THE
GOOD HEALTH
DIRECTORY

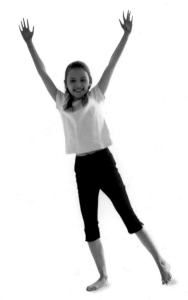

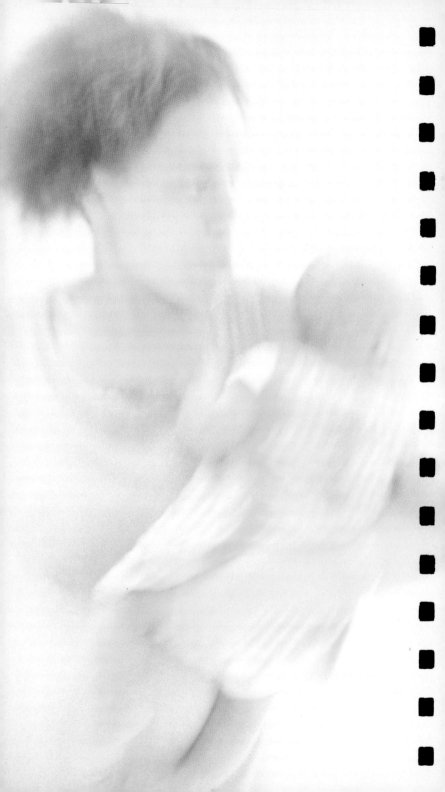

THE
GOOD HEALTH
DIRECTORY

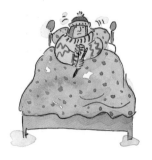

CONSULTANT EDITOR
MICHAEL VAN STRATEN

FOREWORD BY
C. NORMAN SHEALY, M.D., Ph.D.

CONTRIBUTORS
NAOMI CRAFT
JOSIE DRAKE
FIONA DRY
PENELOPE ODY
MICHAEL VAN STRATEN

CONTRIBUTORS

Main introduction, ailment introductions, Kitchen Medicine,
Nutrition, Prevention: MICHAEL VAN STRATEN
Aromatherapy: JOSIE DRAKE
Conventional Medicine: NAOMI CRAFT
Herbal Remedies: PENELOPE ODY
Homeopathic Remedies: FIONA DRY

First edition for the United States, its territories and possessions
published by Barron's Educational Series, Inc. in 2000

Library of Congress Catalog Card Number: 00-101044

ISBN 0-7641-5314-5

All inquiries should be addressed to:
Barron's Educational Series, Inc.
250 Wireless Boulevard, Hauppauge, NY 11788
http://www.barronseduc.com

Note from the publisher
Information given in this book is not intended to be
taken as a replacement for medical advice. Any person
with a condition requiring medical attention should
consult a qualified medical practitioner or therapist.

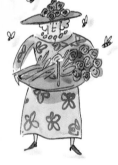

This book was conceived, designed and
produced by
THE IVY PRESS LIMITED
The Old Candlemakers, West Street
Lewes, East Sussex BN7 2NZ

Creative Director: PETER BRIDGEWATER
Designer: JANE LANAWAY
DTP Designer: CHRIS LANAWAY
Editorial Director: DENNY HEMMING
Managing Editor: ANNE TOWNLEY
Editor: MANDY GREENFIELD
Studio Photography: MARIE-LOUISE AVERY,
WALTER GARDINER,
IAN PARSONS, GUY RYECART
Illustrations: MADELEINE HARDIE
Models: MARK JAMIESON
Picture Research: TRUDI VALTER
US Medical Consultant: MELISSA STILES, M.D.,
University of Wisconsin, Madison Department of Family Education

Originated and printed in China by
Hong Kong Graphic and Printing Ltd

9 8 7 6 5 4 3 2 1

Contents

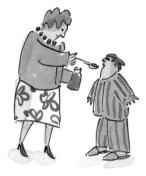

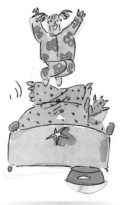

Caution buttons

*The color of the circular button
at the corner of each caution box
indicates the therapy to which
that caution relates:*

🔴 **CONVENTIONAL MEDICINE**

🔴 **HOMEOPATHIC REMEDIES**

🔴 **HERBAL REMEDIES**

🔴 **NUTRITION**

🔴 **AROMATHERAPY**

🔴 **GENERAL WARNING**

Foreword

It has been estimated that well over 90 percent of the improvement in life expectancy in the Western world is the result of four factors: the chlorination of water, adequate sewage disposal, the pasteurization of milk, and adequate calorie intake. Today in the West, however, especially in the United States, we eat too many calories, and that fact alone accounts for many of the diseases that cause premature death. Dr. John Knowles, the late President of the Rockefeller Foundation, estimated that 85 percent of illnesses are actually the result of poor lifestyle choices.

Choosing *good health* habits is the key to preserving your health and quality of life. And when illnesses do occur, you can effectively treat many of them yourself with the safe, time-honored home remedies detailed in this beautifully illustrated book. Of course, many symptoms are beyond the scope of self-treatment and require immediate medical attention. These include sudden severe pain in the head, chest, or abdomen; paralysis or numbness; loss of consciousness; seizures; fever above 102°F in an adult, 103°F in a child under 6; difficulty in breathing; confusion or significant personality changes; an irregular or very rapid heartbeat, or a sudden drop in heart rate below 50 beats per minute; significant swelling or redness of any part of the body; inability to urinate or defecate; significant bleeding; rapid weight loss, especially in conjunction with frequent urination and excessive thirst; a sore that does not heal; change in a wart or mole; frequent indigestion or trouble swallowing; a significant change in bowel habits; a persistent cough or hoarseness; a lump in the breast or scrotum. Any one of these problems should prompt you to see your doctor without delay.

But for symptoms caused by stress that has not yet produced serious damage, you can and should take charge of your own care and treatment. *The Good Health Directory* provides the information and answers you need in order to be both well informed and self reliant.

C. NORMAN SHEALY, M.D., PH.D.

Introduction

There is nothing new about home remedies. From ancient times and in the most primitive of homes, people everywhere have used home remedies to treat everyday ailments and promote good health. Such remedies have been passed down from generation to generation—in the Western world, usually from mother to daughter—and until quite recently, every cookbook featured a section on healing foods.

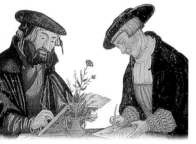

ABOVE Herbalism has been used as a healing therapy for centuries.

From homeopathic remedies for sinusitis to pumpkin seeds for infections and lavender oil for insomnia, *The Good Health Directory* provides effective solutions for dozens of everyday health problems. It tells you not only how to deal with minor ailments, but how to use home remedies to relieve some of the discomforts of complex diseases. All the treatments in the book are the gentle ones that people are seeking these days in order to avoid unnecessary and costly medication with powerful drugs.

The Good Health Directory is organized by body systems, with additional sections on childhood illnesses and first aid. Within each section, you'll find the most common disorders and problems fully described, along with a game plan for treating them with the most effective of the following techniques: conventional medicine, herbal remedies, aromatherapy, nutrition, homeopathic remedies, and in some cases, exercise. The invaluable home pharmacy section at the end of the book provides important background information on the featured techniques, such as how to make your own herbal infusions, tinctures and poultices, the 20 most useful aromatherapeutic oils and healing foods, and the components of a good home medicine chest. Readers new to homeopathy are especially advised to read pages 194–195 in this section and to consult a homeopathic practitioner before using homeopathic remedies on their own.

Many "alternative practitioners" talk about the good old days before we had a pharmaceutical industry, but this is simply living in fantasy land. All treatments and medicines must be viewed in the light of risk and benefit. While it is undoubtedly true that most natural therapies represent minimal risk and valuable benefit, the advances of modern medicine and surgery, as well as the lifesaving benefits of sophisticated pharmaceuticals, cannot be dismissed.

Though many of the remedies in this book are an alternative to other treatments, there is really no such thing as "alternative medicine"—only good and bad medicine. In serious illness, patients are best served by a combination of the most suitable therapies for their particular problems, which is why the term "complementary medicine" is increasingly used. When physicians and other practitioners work together, the patient reaps the greatest benefit.

This book is not meant as a substitute for your physician, though in many instances the safe, simple treatments suggested here will help prevent unnecessary trips to the doctor's office. Remember, though, that first aid is just what it says, and if you are in any doubt as to the seriousness of a symptom—especially when it involves children—then see your physician. Most parents have a natural instinct about the health of their children, and if your gut instinct is worrying you, then do not delay in seeking medical help.

BELOW Children, too, can benefit from treatment with complementary medicines.

Most accidents occur in the home—more than half of us have an accident each year that requires some sort of treatment, and one-fifth of us suffer an injury that requires medical treatment of one kind or another.

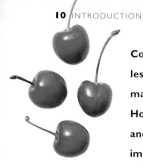

ABOVE Cherries contain vitamin C and bioflavonoids.

Common sense and care can help to make accidents less likely, but it takes a bit more effort to prevent many of the other ailments described in this book. However, making the effort is more than worthwhile, and you will find here detailed advice on how improving your nutrition can help you avoid recurring problems; how aromatherapy can soothe and destress you; and how other home remedies can help boost your resistance to everyday infections.

In today's overcomplicated, technological, and stressful world many of us are eager to take more control of our own lives. Using the home remedies in this book is one step in that direction, and we hope that the information we have provided will give you the self-confidence and the knowledge that you need to tackle many common ailments. Most of the remedies have stood the test of time and can now claim scientific validation. Others are included on the basis of centuries of use and a vast body of anecdotal evidence. Although scientists may scoff, modern medicine has been built on the observations and anecdotes of great practitioners of the healing arts, and some of the most powerful modern drugs were in common use long before clinical trials were even invented.

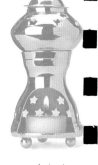

ABOVE A simple vaporizer for burning oils.

We hope that you will quickly discover the many benefits of these simple remedies and, by passing them on to your relatives and friends, will add to the vast body of anecdotal evidence and "old wives' tales" that truly help promote natural good health.

MICHAEL VAN STRATEN

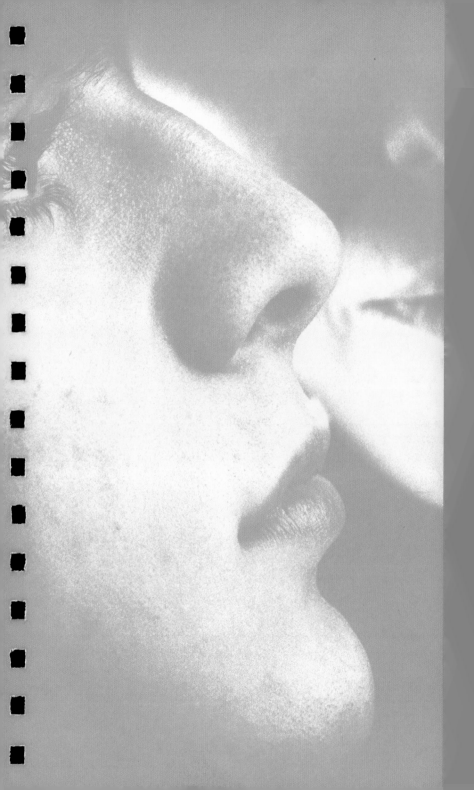

The Immune System

Over the last 20 years or so an inefficient immune system has become the catchall culprit for most day-to-day health problems. Yet few people are aware of the extent to which a healthy lifestyle can strengthen their immune systems, or of how important this body system is in repelling those "ordinary" illnesses that strike all of us from time to time. This section looks at the ills—fever, flu, sore throat, and so on—that can arise from a poorly functioning immune system, and at the best treatments for them, drawn from a variety of disciplines.

Infections: bacterial/viral

Characterized by a fever; other symptoms depend on the underlying cause, but may include muscular aches and pains; shivering; localized soreness and inflammation; sore throat and blocked sinuses.

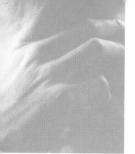

e share the world we live in with teeming billions of bacteria and viruses. **Many have no impact on the human species, some cause minor discomfort, while others cause life-threatening disease. Our natural defense system is a delicate mechanism that needs careful nurturing, and when we ignore its needs we can expect to reap a bitter harvest of ill health, disability, and even death. Nurturing this system starts and finishes in the home.**

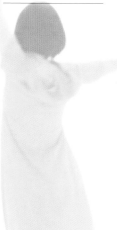

 Call the physician
If very high temperatures, above 102.2°F (39°C), do not respond to conventional medication.

CONVENTIONAL MEDICINE

When you feel feverish, curling up in bed wearing extra clothes may make the problem worse. A warm bath or sponging the body with tepid water will help restore normal body temperature. Wear cool clothing and take a pain reliever. Antibiotics may be prescribed, although viruses will not respond to them.
DOSAGE: ADULTS 1–2 tablets of pain relievers at onset, repeated every 4 hours; consult label.
DOSAGE: CHILDREN Give regular doses of children's pain reliever (do not give aspirin to a child with a fever, due to its link with Reye's syndrome); consult label, or follow medical advice.

HERBAL REMEDIES

Modern research has shown that many herbs can combat viruses or bacteria.
USE AND DOSAGE Echinacea is one of the most effective herbs—take up to 600mg in tablets three times daily at the first sign of infection. (Avoid if you are pregnant or have a disorder of the immune system.)

Garlic is antiviral and antibacterial. Take up to 2g daily in capsules or add 1–2 cloves to cooked dishes.

Chinese tonic herbs, such as shiitake mushrooms, will boost the immune system. Try the mushrooms in soups, or buy them in capsules.

NUTRITION

Building a sound immune system starts three months before conception, with healthy eating by both prospective parents and avoidance of alcohol, large amounts of caffeine, nicotine, and drugs. Optimum nutrition means: a minimum of 5 portions a day of fruit and vegetables; lots of complex carbohydrates such as whole wheat bread, brown rice, pasta, cereals, and beans; a sensible intake of low-fat dairy products; some eggs and at least four portions of oily fish each week; plenty of other fish, poultry, and a little red meat.

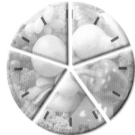

ABOVE Eating 5 portions of fruit and vegetables each day is the basis of a healthy diet.

Good nutrition is important throughout life, but at times of particular stress it is absolutely vital. Get your essential minerals by eating a handful of pumpkin seeds every day for their zinc and five Brazil nuts daily for their selenium. Vitamins A, C, and the all-important E provide a cell protective antioxidant force, while the high natural bacteria content of live yogurt is a great immune-booster.

Caution
Always read pain reliever labels carefully, and do not exceed the stated dose.

AROMATHERAPY

- Tea tree *(Melaleuca alternifolia)*
- Lavender *(Lavandula angustifolia)*
- Thyme *(Thymus vulgaris)*
- Niaouli *(Melaleuca viridiflora)*
- Bergamot *(Citrus bergamia)*

All of these oils attack infectious organisms, kill airborne germs, and strengthen the body's immune system.

APPLICATION Depends on what is most convenient or pleasant for the user.

HOMEOPATHIC REMEDIES

In homeopathy the patient is treated according to symptoms that the body produces, and not necessarily according to the type of infection that leads to those symptoms *(so look at Fever on p.16, Influenza on p.18, Sore throat on p.20, etc.).*

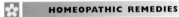

THYME

Allergies

*Characterized by sneezing fits, red and itchy eyes, itchy skin, a
runny nose, and congested nasal passages; more severe
symptoms may include wheezing, difficulty in swallowing, and
swollen lips and tongue.*

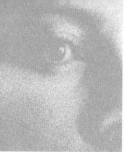

BELOW Wearing
a medical allergy
necklace can
save your life.

An allergy is an **exaggerated response by the
body's natural defense mechanisms, very
often to something that would not normally be a hazard. The body wrongly identifies a food, a pollen, or an
atmospheric pollutant as a dangerous invader; the white
cells overreact; and this "allergic response" then becomes an
illness in itself. Sometimes avoidance of the allergen is the only
cure; but home remedies can make an enormous difference.**

LEFT Nasal
sprays can
bring some
relief from
allergies for
both adults
and children.

Caution

*Violent allergic
reactions—
anaphylaxis—can be
fatal. Sufferers should
carry an emergency
injection of adrenalin.
Breathing difficulties
or swelling of the
face constitute
dire emergencies.*

✚ CONVENTIONAL MEDICINE

Mild symptoms can be treated with antihistamines
or steroid nose drops. For more severe allergic
reactions, such as some cases of peanut allergy, seek
urgent medical attention. If you know you have a
severe allergic reaction, wear a MedicAlert bracelet
or necklace describing your allergy.

DOSAGE: ADULTS Antihistamines are available as
tablets, syrup, or eyedrops; some preparations can
cause drowsiness. Most tablets are taken once a
day; eyedrops more frequently—consult label for
details, or follow medical advice. Apply 2 puffs of
nose spray per nostril twice a day.

DOSAGE: CHILDREN Doses of antihistamine syrup
depend on the age of the child; consult your pharmacist, read the label for details, or follow medical
advice. Apply 2 puffs of nose spray per nostril
twice a day to children over six.

✤ HOMEOPATHIC REMEDIES

There are many homeopathic remedies which
address allergies, but treatment depends on individualizing the nature of the symptom; visit a qualified
homeopath for an accurate prescription. (See also
p. 194, Congestion on p.42, and Hay fever on p.48.)

NUTRITION

Foods are among the commonest causes of allergic reactions, either through eating them or through contact (see Dermatitis on p.132). Allergies often run in families, but there is evidence that exposure to some foods too early in life (such as cow's milk or peanuts) can also cause problems. The most common food allergens are milk, eggs, dairy products, shellfish, nuts, berries, wheat, and corn. But allergies—very rapid reactions to minute amounts of the culprit—should not be confused with food intolerance, which produces symptoms hours after consumption. Milk intolerance is a very common problem, whereas true milk allergy is quite rare.

All foods that are rich in B vitamins can help reduce the severity of allergic symptoms, and oily fish can help in treating eczema, due to its high content of omega-3 fatty acids.

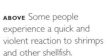

ABOVE Some people experience a quick and violent reaction to shrimps and other shellfish.

Caution
Several herbs, particularly fresh rue, can trigger allergic reactions. If using true melissa, which is very rare and expensive, be very careful about how you use it, for it can cause nasty burns to the skin.

HERBAL REMEDIES

Garlic is traditionally used to combat food allergies— add cloves to cooking or take garlic capsules daily. Regular cups of agrimony tea can improve the digestive system's ability to cope with allergens, while marigold will help combat the fungal infections often associated with food allergy. Teas made from chamomile, elder, or yarrow flowers can also reduce allergic reactions.

GARLIC CAPSULES

BELOW Marigold is useful for fighting the fungal infections that occur with food allergies.

AROMATHERAPY

- Melissa *(Melissa officinalis)*
- Roman chamomile *(Chamaemelum nobile)*
- Lavender *(Lavandula angustifolia)*

These oils soothe and relax the body after its over-reaction to the external stimulus. They are also calming to the emotions.

APPLICATION This will depend on the form that the allergy takes. If there is irritation on the skin, use a compress, soothing baths, or a lotion containing a few drops of the oils, which can be rubbed in regularly. If the skin is too irritated to be touched, use a spray.

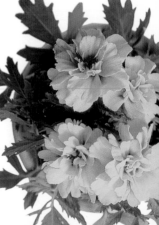

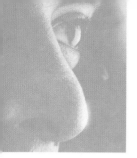

Fever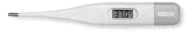

Classic fever symptoms include shivering and a hot, dry skin as the body temperature rises; there may also be aching limbs and copious perspiration, accompanied by a considerable thirst.

A fever or high temperature is the body's way of reacting to an attack by invading bacteria or viruses. The body's temperature is strictly regulated and is normally between 98.4° and 99.5°F (36.9° and 37.5°C). As little as half-a-degree change in temperature may make you feel unwell and suggests there is an infection somewhere in the body. In most cases, the problem is self-limiting, and the normal sort of high temperature caused by a flu, for example, may be left to run its course. However, a very high temperature or a prolonged bout of fever for which there is no obvious cause requires immediate medical attention.

 Call the physician

If very high temperatures, above 102.2°F (39°C), do not respond to conventional medication; are accompanied by cystitis, headache or abdominal pain; or persist for more than 24 hours.

 CONVENTIONAL MEDICINE

Curling up under blankets when you feel shivery and unwell can raise the body temperature and make the problem worse. Try a warm bath or sponging the body with tepid water. Dress in cool clothing and take a pain reliever. Antibiotics may be prescribed to treat the cause of the fever.

DOSAGE: ADULTS 1–2 tablets of pain relievers at onset of fever, repeated every 4 hours; consult label for details.

DOSAGE: CHILDREN Give regular doses of children's pain reliever (do not give aspirin to a child with a fever, due to its link with Reye's syndrome); consult label for details, or follow medical advice.

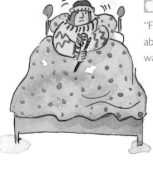

 NUTRITION

"Feed a cold and starve a fever"—the old adage is absolutely correct. You will not feel like eating any-way, but the body will lose huge amounts of fluid through sweating, so copious drinks are essen-tial: diluted fresh citrus juices for their immune-boosting vitamin C; pineapple juice for its soothing enzymes (cartons of juice are fine); and herbal teas—particularly chamomile and elderflower. To keep your immune system working efficiently, ensure a regular intake of vitamin C, zinc, selenium, and all the carotenoids by eating a wide variety of fruits and vegetables, nuts and seeds.

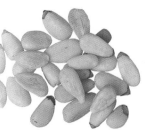

ABOVE Nuts of all kinds can help to boost the immune system.

✿ HOMEOPATHIC REMEDIES

There are many homeopathic remedies indicated, but these are among the most common.

☜ Aconite 30c

For first stage of illness. If no improvement try:

☜ Belladonna 30c

For rapid onset, high fever, red burning face, dry skin, cold feet. Dilated pupils.

☜ Gelsemium 30c

For heavy, aching limbs. Drowsy, chills up and down spine. **DOSAGE** 1 tablet every 30 minutes, for six doses, then every 4 hours. Maximum 3 days.

💧 AROMATHERAPY

☜ **Roman chamomile** (*Chamaemelum nobile*)
☜ **Lavender** (*Lavandula angustifolia*)
☜ **Tea tree** (*Melaleuca alternifolia*)
☜ **Juniper** (*Juniperus communis*)
☜ **Peppermint** (*Mentha x piperita*)

Tea tree and juniper (avoid if you are pregnant or have a kidney problem) encourage the body to sweat if it needs to eliminate excess fluid. Avoid peppermint if you have a gallbladder or liver problem. Chamomile is soothing.

APPLICATION Use either in a bath or in low doses in cool water, to sponge the body down.

🌿 HERBAL REMEDIES

Herbs have long been used in fever management—cooling the body during the "hot" stages by encouraging sweating (e.g. with yarrow, lime flowers, boneset) and stimulating the digestion (using bitters such as gentian or wormwood), then heating the system during the "chill" stage (with stimulants like angelica or ginger—do not use if you have gallstones).

USE AND DOSAGE Confine home remedies to milder case, using appropriate herbal infusions (see p.186).

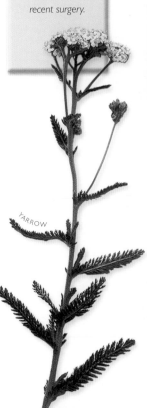

Caution

Be particularly alert for fevers starting after trips abroad, after accidents involving cuts and grazes, contact with animals, or recent surgery.

YARROW

Influenza

High fever; headache, joint pains, general muscular aches and pains;, fatigue and lack of energy, often accompanied by a loss of appetite, sneezing; sore throat and a dry cough; swollen glands in the neck.

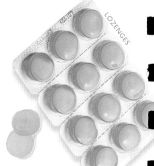

This is an acute viral infection that recurs throughout the population every year. Approximately every three years flu reaches epidemic proportions, as new strains of virus appear to which the general population has no acquired immunity. So make sure that your kitchen cupboard is always equipped with the necessary home remedies.

Call the physician

If a cough is getting worse and you are finding it difficult to breathe.

BELOW Drink plenty of fluids during a bout of flu, especially when you have no appetite for food.

CONVENTIONAL MEDICINE

Influenza is caused by a virus infection and will not respond to antibiotics. Shivers and muscular aches can be eased by taking pain relievers, while lozenges and hot drinks can help to soothe a sore throat. Rest in bed and drink plenty of water. Some strains of influenza can be warded off by annual vaccination.

DOSAGE: ADULTS 1–2 tablets of pain relievers at onset, repeated every 4 hours; consult label for details.

DOSAGE: CHILDREN Give regular doses of children's pain reliever (do not give aspirin to a child with a fever, due to its link with Reye's syndrome); consult label, or follow medical advice.

HOMEOPATHIC REMEDIES

There are many homeopathic remedies indicated, but these are among the most common.

Gelsemium 30c

For drowsiness. Head heavy. Chills up and down spine. No thirst. Trembling legs. Muscular soreness.

Eupatorium perfoliatum 30c

For pain in bones and aching muscles. Thirsty. Throbbing headache. Aches better for sweating.

DOSAGE 1 tablet every 4 hours until improved. Maximum 12 doses.

HERBAL REMEDIES

Herbs can help to relieve flu's symptoms, as well as combat the debilitation that often follows an attack. **USE AND DOSAGE** Mix equal amounts of boneset, yarrow, elderflower, and peppermint (avoid if you have a gallbladder or liver problem) and make an infusion with 2tsp per cup.

A compress soaked in lavender tea will ease feverish headaches.

As a post-flu tonic, combine a decoction of ele-campane root with an equal amount of an infusion of vervain and St. John's wort.

NUTRITION

The time to worry about nutrition and flu is before you get it. So boost your immune system by follow-ing the advice given under Infection (see p.12). If you do catch flu, rest and return to regular activity slowly and as tolerated. For the first 24 hours, drink plenty of fluids: lots of soothing lemon juice, hot water, and honey (but not for children under two), as well as pineapple juice for its healing enzymes; eat only grapes, berries, citrus fruits, and ripe pears. The next day, add cooked vegetables. On the third day, add bread, potatoes, rice, and pasta. By day four, you can resume your normal diet.

CRANBERRIES

During a bout of flu, take 1g of vitamin C three times a day, 5,000 IU of vitamin A, and a high-strength B-complex supplement. After a week, reduce the dose to 1g of vitamin C each day, 1,000 IU of vitamin A, and the B-complex supple-ment; continue for at least 3 weeks.

AROMATHERAPY

~ **Tea tree** (*Melaleuca alternifolia*)
Tea tree will make you sweat, which should help alleviate symptoms.
APPLICATION Put 4–6 drops into a warm bath and soak; drink a large glass of water and go to bed. Use steam inhalations and burners to stop cross infection and to treat symptoms.

> **Caution**
> *Flu can be complicated by secondary chest infections and possibly pneumonia. The very young, the elderly, and anyone with asthma, chronic bronchitis, other chronic respiratory diseases, heart disease, kidney problems, diabetes, or a suppressed immune system should get medical help for flu at once.*

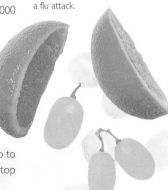

BELOW Grapes and citrus fruits should be eaten during the early stages of a flu attack.

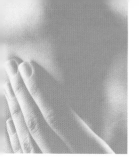

Sore throat

Characterized by a scratchy pain in the throat; a sore cough, or a hoarse, sore voice; it may follow a cold, overusing the voice, or breathing in smoke; sometimes linked to tonsillitis (see p.158).

A sore throat (pharyngitis) may be caused by a viral infection, dehydration, overuse of the voice or shouting (laryngitis), or it may be an early symptom of other infectious diseases. It can also be caused by infection, inflammation and/or enlargement of the tonsils. Sore throats are common and uncomfortable, but they are usually of little clinical significance.

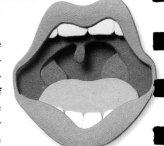

ABOVE A sore throat should not generally last for more than a week or so.

🌐 Call the physician

If there is any change in the quality of your voice that does not return to normal within a week or two; if you have been hoarse for a period of more than 6 weeks.

✚ CONVENTIONAL MEDICINE

Sore vocal cords need rest. Steam inhalations *(see p.196)* can help to reduce the swelling around the cords; use as often as needed. Cough syrups or lozenges may help.

DOSAGE: ADULTS 1–2 spoonfuls of cough syrup or 1 lozenge every 4–5 hours; consult label for details, or follow medical advice.

DOSAGE: CHILDREN 1 spoonful of cough syrup or half a lozenge three times daily; consult label for details, or follow medical advice.

HERBAL REMEDIES

Soothing, astringent, and antiseptic herbs for use in gargles include sage, myrrh, lady's mantle, thyme, potentilla, and agrimony. (Avoid sage if you are pregnant or breastfeeding).

USE AND DOSAGE Make a strong infusion (2–3tsp per cup), strain well, and gargle every 30–60 minutes while symptoms persist. Fresh *Aloe vera* sap added to the gargle will also help (avoid if pregnant or you have a bowel disorder; not for children under 12). Drink a standard infusion (1tsp per cup) of any of the above herbs as well.

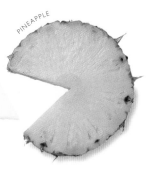

PINEAPPLE

 ## NUTRITION

For an acute sore throat, especially with a fever, a 24-hour raw fruit and fruit-juice fast will boost the immune system and provide essential nutrients. Drink plenty of pineapple juice and citrus juices diluted 50:50 with water; eat lots of avocados, together with exotic fruits, like pineapple, papaya (avoid if pregnant), and mango. If you are prescribed antibiotics, make sure you have plenty of live yogurt to recondition the natural bacteria in your intestines. But the throat's best friend is the kitchen faucet: 4–6 glasses of water each day are essential, together with other drinks. And hot water with 2 tsp of honey (not for children under two) and the juice of half a lemon is a most soothing remedy.

HOMEOPATHIC REMEDIES

Belladonna 30c
For sudden onset. Throat red, dry, painful, initially on right side. Swallowing very painful.

Phytolacca 30c
For pain in ears on swallowing. Swallowing hot drinks impossible. Dark red tonsils, right side especially swollen. Neck stiff.

Lachesis 30c
For left-sided pain initially, spreading to right. Sensation of tightness in throat, sensitive to touch. Wakes with sore throat. Difficult to swallow saliva, worse for hot drinks.

DOSAGE 1 tablet every 2 hours for six doses, followed by every 4 hours until improved. Maximum 12 doses.

AROMATHERAPY

Sandalwood (Santalum album)
Myrrh (Commiphora molmol)
Tea tree (Melaleuca alternifolia)
These are antibacterial, fungicidal, and help kill pain. Avoid sandalwood if you have a kidney problem.
APPLICATION Put the oils into a massage oil or cream and use them on the throat area. Then wrap something warm around the throat.

Caution
Recurrent and chronic sore throats may be caused by smoking, excessive alcohol use, repeated vomiting (as in bulimia), or even by a hiatal hernia.

Prevention
To protect your throat, keep your salt consumption to a minimum, drink only modest amounts of alcohol (not spirits), stop smoking, and avoid very hot drinks and cola drinks, which irritate the throat's delicate membranes.

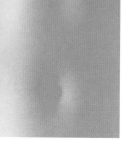

Shingles

A burning sensation felt on an area of sensitive skin, which then develops blisters; it most commonly affects an area around the shoulder, chest, or waist, or one side of the face and one eye.

hingles (*Herpes zoster* is its medical name) is caused by the same virus that causes chicken pox. After chicken pox, some of the virus stays dormant in nerve ganglions for many years. Later in life, a weakening of the immune system—due to stress, illness, advancing age, or immunosuppressant drugs—can reactivate the virus, causing shingles. Up to 20 percent of adults are affected, but the elderly and those with a suppressed immune system are at greatest risk. For some, shingles is a mild infection; it leaves others with a very painful condition called "post-herpetic neuralgia," which may persist for months or even years.

 Call the physician
If you think you are suffering from shingles.

BELOW Elderly people can be particularly susceptible to shingles.

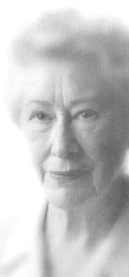

 CONVENTIONAL MEDICINE

If you develop symptoms of shingles you may need treatment from your physician. Contact your doctor immediately if shingles affects your eye; it could cause permanent damage. Antiviral drugs are only effective if given early, as soon as the rash erupts. Strong pain relievers will also help.

HERBAL REMEDIES

Shingles is a condition that responds to a variety of herbal remedies.

USE AND DOSAGE During an attack, echinacea (up to 2g in tablets daily; avoid if you are pregnant or have a disorder of the immune system) will help to combat the viral infection.

Drinking plenty of St. John's wort infusion may limit the risk of lingering nerve pain.

A tea containing equal amounts of passion flower, lemon balm, and wild lettuce will also ease the pain and discomfort.

Apply fresh *Aloe vera* sap to any blistering that occurs. Afterward, use vervain or St. John's wort in either creams or infused oils in order to combat nerve pain.

AROMATHERAPY

- Eucalyptus *(Eucalyptus radiata)*
- Tea tree *(Melaleuca alternifolia)*
- Lavender *(Lavandula angustifolia)*
- Roman chamomile *(Chamaemelum nobile)*
- Bergamot *(Citrus bergamia)*

These oils are painkilling, antiviral, and help to dry out the blisters. Bergamot is active against the *Herpes zoster* virus. Tea-tree oil also helps to build up the body's immune system. Do not use eucalyptus if you have digestive problems or liver disease; do not give to infants or small children.

APPLICATION Smooth the oils very gently over the affected area and down either side of the spine, where all the nerve endings are. If the body is too painful to touch, add the oils to a water spray; use a very soft brush to paint the oils on; or use the oils in the bath.

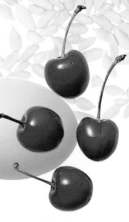

ABOVE Eating cherries, eggs, and seeds will help to boost your nutrient levels.

NUTRITION

The B vitamins, bioflavonoids, and vitamin C are the key nutrients, so eat plenty of citrus fruits, together with some of the pith and skin between the segments; dark cherries, tomatoes, and mangoes; eggs, poultry, and liver; nuts, seeds, and whole wheat cereals; olive, sunflower, and safflower oils. Do not forget that the probiotic bacteria that are present in live yogurt are an essential factor in the body's production of some B vitamins.

HOMEOPATHIC REMEDIES

- Rhus toxicodendron 6c

For painful, small, watery blisters with a lot of itching. Better for warm applications. Person is restless, which helps to relieve itching. Probably the most common remedy for shingles.

- Ranunculus bulbosus 6c

For burning pain, itching worse for touch. Bluish appearance of spots, which appear in clusters. Neuralgia of the chest wall.

DOSAGE 1 tablet every 4 hours until blisters have settled. Maximum 5 days.

Prevention

Improved nutrition and supplements may help to prevent attacks. It may be useful to take a small dose (0.5g) of the essential amino acid L-lysine, plus a vitamin B-complex.

Caution

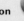

Shingles that affects the eye may cause serious complications and should be monitored carefully by your physician.

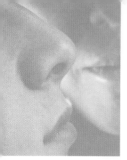

Cold Sores:
herpes simplex

An itchy or sore area, usually around the mouth or nose; a cluster of small blisters, which may ooze clear fluid before crusting over.

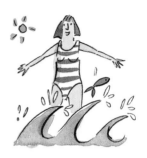

These unsightly, uncomfortable skin eruptions, which are caused by the *Herpes simplex* virus, may be the result of a cold, but are triggered by stress—physical or emotional. Women often get cold sores during their periods; vacationers when exposed to too much sun.

 Call the physician

If you suffer from recurrent herpes.

BELOW Cold sores are not serious but can make you feel uncomfortable and miserable.

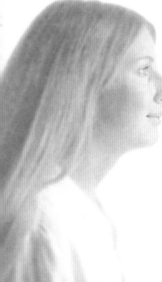

 CONVENTIONAL MEDICINE

Creams containing antiviral drugs, available only by prescription, may limit minor outbreaks, if used early. Antiviral tablets, available only by prescription, help prevent frequent recurrences and limit severe attacks.

DOSAGE: ADULTS Take tablets up to five times a day for 5 days: follow medical advice; creams more often.

DOSAGE: CHILDREN Follow medical advice given for tablets. Apply creams every few hours.

 HERBAL REMEDIES

Tea-tree oil, lavender oil, and clove oil, *Aloe vera* sap, calendula cream, sliced garlic, and house-leek juice can all help to alleviate the discomfort caused by cold sores.

USE AND DOSAGE Capsules containing goldenseal, echinacea, or nettle help combat the infection. (Avoid if you are pregnant or breastfeeding.)

 HOMEOPATHIC REMEDIES

This is the most common homeopathic remedy.

🐌 **Natrum muriaticum 6c**

For pearly white sores. May have mouth ulcers, burning of lower lip. Dry mouth. Cracks in lower lip.

DOSAGE 1 tablet every 4 hours. Maximum 1 week.

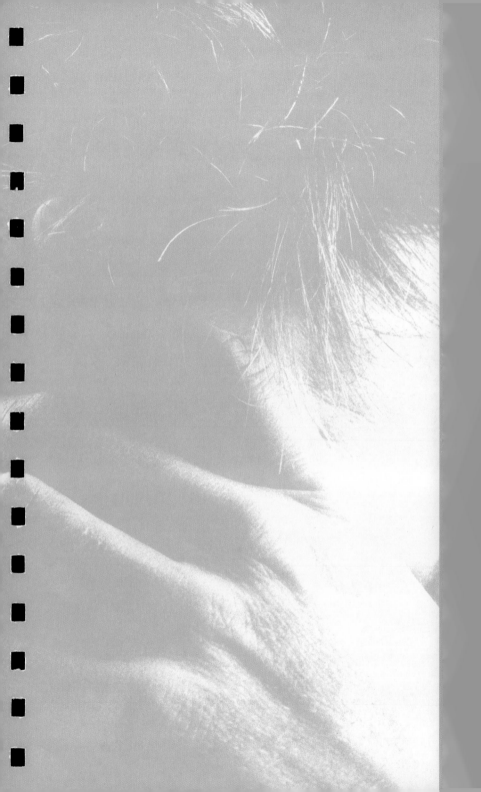

The Nervous System

The nervous system is an ultra-complex organization of nerves that carries impulses throughout the body, from organs such as the ears and eyes, skin and joints, to the brain. This delicate system is easily upset, leading to fatigue, stress, headaches, and insomnia. Simple home remedies, however, can greatly relieve many of these ailments. Food, for example, has long been seen as nourishment not only for the body but also for the mind, while aromatherapy—smell being the most primitive of our senses—has a direct effect on the brain.

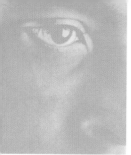

Neuralgia

Pain that is experienced like a knife or electric shock, often felt on one side of the face, where the trigeminal nerve is affected (trigeminal neuralgia); it may then settle down into a continual ache; other parts of the body are also vulnerable.

euralgia is nerve tissue pain, usually felt at the ends of the nervous system—that is, near the surface of the skin. The most common forms are postherpetic neuralgia (which often follows a bout of shingles; see p.22) and trigeminal neuralgia. These can both be so excruciating that washing, shaving, and even the weight of sheets may be unbearable. In the treatment of neuralgia home remedies are not hugely successful, but neither are the very powerful drugs that are normally prescribed. The best chance of success comes from a combination of orthodox treatment, acupuncture, and self-help.

BELOW Neuralgia can be stinging pain, soreness, tingling, or numbness.

CONVENTIONAL MEDICINE

Warmth or massage may help during an attack. Pain relievers may not be sufficient to control the pain, and your physician may prescribe drugs used in other patients to treat depression or epilepsy. In intractable cases your physician can refer you to a pain clinic, where a specialist may recommend a combination of different treatments, including behavioral therapy and acupuncture.

DOSAGE: ADULTS 1–2 tablets of pain relievers at onset of pain, repeated every 4 hours; consult label.

DOSAGE: CHILDREN Give regular doses of children's pain reliever; consult label, or follow medical advice.

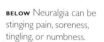 HERBAL REMEDIES

Smooth warmed lemon juice or diluted lemon oil on the painful area. Cayenne creams and oil are also useful externally, especially if the pain follows shingles (may cause a burning sensation, do not use on broken skin; avoid if pregnant); internally, herbs to help repair nerves can be useful.

USE AND DOSAGE Drink a combination of St. John's wort, vervain, and chamomile (equal amounts, 2tsp of the mix per cup).

NUTRITION

Eat plenty of potatoes, liver (but not if you are pregnant), nuts and seeds, brown rice, Brazil nuts, milk, eggs, poultry, whole wheat bread, dried fruits, green and root vegetables, legumes, and fish for their B vitamins, which are essential in the diet of neuralgia sufferers. If chewing is painful, make some soup from a wide variety of the foods containing the B vitamins, so that it can be drunk from a cup or, if this is easier, through a thick straw. Old-fashioned, homemade chicken soup enriched with barley and brown rice offers a simple, nutritious and delicious way of providing B vitamins.

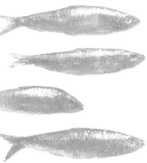

ABOVE All types of fish contain the essential B vitamins.

HOMEOPATHIC REMEDIES

Spigelia 6c
For left-sided pain, like hot needles, sharp. Pain above left eye—person can point to the spot. Pain worse for stooping or opening mouth.

Causticum 6c
For right-sided facial neuralgia, burning pain. Worse for wind and for change of weather. Pain in jaws, worse for opening mouth.

Aconite 6c
For use in first stages. Intense pain after going out in cold, dry wind. Often left-sided. May have tingling and numbness.

DOSAGE 1 tablet hourly for six doses, then every 4–6 hours. Maximum 3 days.

> **Caution**
> Do not use rosemary oil if you have high blood pressure.

AROMATHERAPY

Lavender (Lavandula angustifolia)
Roman chamomile (Chamaemelum nobile)
Marjoram (Origanum majorana)
Rosemary (Rosmarinus officinalis)

These oils help to ease the pain and tension of neuralgia. (Avoid rosemary if pregnant; do not give marjoram to babies or small children.)

APPLICATION They are best used in a cold compress held over the affected area. Do be aware that neuralgia is aggravated by stress (see p.36), so also find an antistress oil that you can use in the bath.

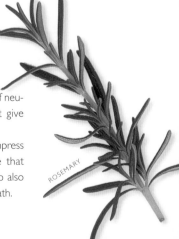

ROSEMARY

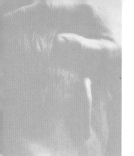

Headaches

Headache all over the scalp, with pain in the neck and shoulder muscles—likely causes: stress, tension, poor posture; frontal headache—likely causes: eyestrain, sinusitis; throbbing one-sided headache with nausea—likely cause: migraine.

eadaches are one of the most common reasons for consulting a physician, yet they are rarely a symptom of any underlying disease. Though they frequently accompany acute infections, many routine headaches are mechanical in origin. Stress, anxiety, hormonal changes, poor posture, badly designed work stations, and the ever-growing use of computers can all result in tension developing in the neck and shoulders: by far the most common cause of everyday headaches.

Caution
Always read pain reliever labels carefully, and do not exceed the stated dose.

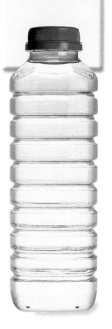

 CONVENTIONAL MEDICINE

Drink plenty of water. Have a warm bath to relieve the tension. Rest in a quiet, darkened room and take a pain reliever.

DOSAGE: ADULTS 1–2 tablets of pain relievers at onset of pain, then every 4 hours; consult label.

DOSAGE: CHILDREN Give regular doses of children's nonaspirin pain reliever; consult label, or follow medical advice.

NUTRITION

Low blood-sugar levels can trigger headaches. Eat at least some whole wheat toast and a banana for breakfast. Always have a banana and a bag of nuts and dried fruits to nibble on throughout the day. Beware of sudden drastic changes in your eating patterns; very low-calorie diets will also cause headaches, as will excessive alcohol and caffeine. A low fluid intake is a common causes of headaches. Drink at least 4 glasses of water every day, as well as other drinks. Because some foods can trigger migraines, it's important to differentiate between ordinary headaches and migraine *(see p.30).*

LEFT Boost your intake of fluids if you are prone to headaches.

HERBAL REMEDIES

There are various relaxing herbs for headaches.
Use and Dosage Tension headaches often respond
to betony and skullcap tea (1tsp of each per cup).

Use rosemary or a low dose of Korean ginseng
(200mg daily) for headaches associated with
overexertion and tiredness. Avoid both if pregnant.

For headaches with depression use a combination of oats and vervain (1tsp of each per cup).

Lavender is good for burning headaches—use a
few drops of undiluted tincture on the tongue or
drink an infusion.

AROMATHERAPY

- Lavender *(Lavandula angustifolia)*
- Peppermint *(Mentha x piperita)*
- Eucalyptus *(Eucalyptus radiata)*
- Basil *(Ocimum basilicum)*

Lavender is calming, soothing, and a natural
painkiller. Peppermint (avoid if you have a gallbladder or liver problem) and basil (avoid if pregnant)
clear the head. Eucalyptus clears the sinuses, but do
not use if you have digestive problems or liver disease; do not give to infants or small children.

Application Put the oil on a facecloth with some
cool water and use as a compress. For headaches,
massage a drop of neat lavender into the temples; a
steam inhalation with eucalyptus will also help

HOMEOPATHIC REMEDIES

There are many homeopathic remedies indicated,
but these are among the most common.

- Bryonia 30c

For pressing, bursting, or splitting headache over left
eye. Pain worse for least movement (even of the
eye), for light, cough, or stooping. Better for pressure.

- Colubrina 30c

For splitting or "hangover" headache, sore scalp, dizziness. Better for warmth, lying down. Worse for
movement, drafts. Person is irritable, oversensitive.

Dosage 1 tablet every 4 hours, as needed.
Maximum six doses.

 Call the physician

*If the headache is
the result of a blow to
the head; if there is
numbness, confusion, or
sudden drowsiness; if you
have a headache and
fever together with pain
on bending forward, stiff
neck, nausea, or a dislike
of bright light; if a very
severe headache starts
suddenly; if your balance,
speech, memory, or vision
is affected; if you wake
up with headaches that
are worse when you
cough or sneeze.*

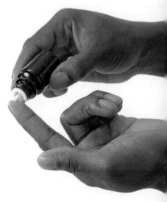

ABOVE A dab of lavender
oil on the fingertips can
be massaged into the
temples for relief from
many types of headache.

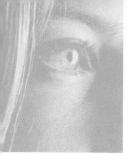

Migraine

Severe headache, which often starts with distorted vision; pain is frequently throbbing, on one side of the head, near an eye, and associated with nausea or vomiting; there may be pins and needles or weakness during an attack.

I t is common for people who suffer from regular headaches to describe them as migraines. Sadly, there is no mistaking a real migraine, with its visual disturbances, nausea, violent vomiting and blinding pain. There is now a wide variety of drug treatments for migraine, but self-help may be the best long-term key to success. Hormonal changes can play a role in migraine. This type of headache is far more common in women than in men, especially around their periods: migraines tend to start after puberty and may improve after the menopause. It is common for migraine to run in families.

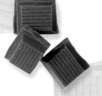

ABOVE AND BELOW Watch your diet to spot any foods or drinks that trigger your migraine.

 CONVENTIONAL MEDICINE

Over-the-counter pain relievers may ease a mild attack. Many prescription drugs are available to abort or even prevent attacks. Lie down in a darkened room, if possible, and drink plenty of water.

DOSAGE: ADULTS 1–2 tablets of pain relievers at onset of pain, repeated every 4 hours; consult label.

DOSAGE: CHILDREN Give regular doses of children's pain reliever; consult label, or follow medical advice.

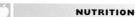 **NUTRITION**

Naturopaths have known for decades that there is a link between migraine and food. The most common triggers are chocolate, citrus fruits, cheese, and caffeine, though red and fortified wine, yeast extracts, pickled herrings, sauerkraut, and other fermented foods are also thought to be causes. Many of these contain the chemical tyramine, which irritates blood vessels in the brain. Two or three glasses of cold water at the very earliest signs of a migraine may be enough to abort an attack, while ginger tea (see *Motion Sickness on p.184*) can help prevent vomiting, but it must be taken at the first sign of an attack and avoid ginger if you have gallstones.

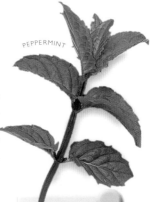

PEPPERMINT

 HERBAL REMEDIES

Lavender and betony are useful migraine herbs.
USE AND DOSAGE Combine equal amounts of both herbs in an infusion and sip while the pain continues.

Add 10 drops of feverfew tincture to a little water and take at 15-minute intervals during a migraine attack. (Do not give to children under 12.)

Evening primrose oil and other good sources of essential fatty acids (cold water fish, hempseed oil) help prevent blood vessels from constricting.

 AROMATHERAPY

- Lavender *(Lavandula angustifolia)*
- Melissa *(Melissa officinalis)*
- Peppermint *(Mentha x piperita)* [if the migraine is accompanied by nausea and vomiting]

Lavender is calming, soothing, and a natural painkiller. Peppermint clears the head and stimulates the brain (avoid if you have a gallbladder or liver problem). Melissa is anti-depressive and gently sedative.

APPLICATION Put the oil on a facecloth with some cool water and use as a compress on the forehead or the back of the neck. Add peppermint or melissa to the lavender or use them separately. Alternatively, put a drop of undiluted lavender on the tips of your fingers and massage well into the temples.

HOMEOPATHIC REMEDIES

It is often best to consult a qualified homeopath for the treatment of migraine.

- Iris 30c

For blurred vision or visual disturbances, then right-sided headache with nausea. Better for gentle motion. Often occurs on weekends.

- Sanguinaria 30c

For pulsating headache, beginning at back of head and extending to right eye. Better for burping and vomiting, being asleep. Worse for light, noise, fasting. Starts in morning, improving during the day.

DOSAGE 1 tablet every 30 minutes until improved. Maximum six doses.

> ### Caution
> Avoid feverfew if you're pregnant or taking prescribed blood-thinning drugs such as warfarin or heparin, as it can reduce the blood's clotting ability still further.

> ### Prevention
> Keep a detailed food and drink diary for at least 3 weeks. Then go back and identify foods eaten up to 3 hours before an attack. This will guide you toward foods that you should eliminate from your diet.

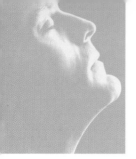

Fatigue

Characterized by either mental or physical exhaustion; sleeping for longer than usual and waking feeling tired; an inability to concentrate and difficulty in summoning up the effort to rectify the problem.

Extreme fatigue has become a problem of almost epidemic proportions in both the US and Britain, but it should not be confused with chronic fatigue syndrome or ME *(see p.34)*, in which fatigue is just one symptom of a more complex illness. In treating extreme fatigue, it is important to rule out the presence of any underlying complaint, such as anemia, thyroid problems, diabetes, or mononucleosis. In the absence of a more specific diagnosis, extreme fatigue is most likely to be caused by stress, poor nutrition, insomnia *(see p.38)*, snoring, sleep apnea, anxiety, or depression.

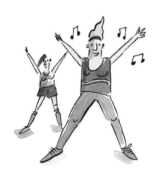

 CONVENTIONAL MEDICINE

Try to sleep regularly for 7–9 hours a night. Take regular exercise and eat a balanced diet, avoiding excessive alcohol. Consider taking some time out from domestic or paid employment. If symptoms persist for more than 2 weeks, see your physician, who may arrange for some blood tests to rule out a physical cause for your symptoms. Avoid aspirin.

NUTRITION

A full complement of the many essential nutrients is the first requirement, and this can only be achieved by a well-balanced diet.

Rich sources of iron, like liver (in limited quantities or not at all if you're pregnant), dates, raisins, watercress, eggs, dark green leafy vegetables, and sardines, must top your shopping list. Eat plenty of foods rich in vitamin C alongside the iron-rich foods to improve absorption—tomatoes with the sardines, orange juice with your boiled eggs.

Avoid all the commercial energy drinks, and do not go overboard on protein. Eat good quality foods rich in complex carbohydrates—not cookies, cakes, and candies. Go for small amounts of meat, plenty of whole grains (e.g. brown rice, whole

 Call the physician

If your symptoms have been present for more than 2 weeks.

wheat pasta), and lots of vegetables or salad. It is especially important to keep blood-sugar levels on a constantly even keel, and this can be best achieved by eating little and often. An effective plan is to eat good-quality foods at least every 3 hours. Nuts, seeds, cereals, and dried fruits are excellent sources of energy.

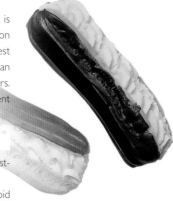

 HERBAL REMEDIES

Herbal tonics can be extremely effective in boosting energy levels to combat fatigue.

USE AND DOSAGE Korean ginseng (600mg daily, avoid if pregnant) is popular but can prove too stimulating for many—traditionally, it has been recommended only for older people (40-plus). American ginseng is gentler; women may prefer Dong Quai (avoid both if pregnant). Take Siberian ginseng (600mg daily) during busy times to help cope with additional stresses.

ABOVE Boost your starch intake, but ensure that you make healthy choices.

 AROMATHERAPY

- Rosemary *(Rosmarinus officinalis)*
- Lemon grass *(Cymbopogon citratus)*
- Basil *(Ocimum basilicum)*
- Peppermint *(Mentha x piperita)*

Rosemary, basil (avoid rosemary and basil if pregnant), and peppermint (avoid if you have a gallbladder or liver problem) stimulate the brain.

APPLICATION Use these oils in the bath, in massage oils or lotions, in vaporizers, or on a handkerchief.

Prevention

Regular supplementation with zinc and a daily iron supplement should be routine for anyone on antidepressants or tranquilizers. Co-enzyme Q10 is another link in the conversion of food-to-energy chain and should also be taken every day.

 HOMEOPATHIC REMEDIES

A consultation with a qualified homeopath is recommended for fatigue. There are many remedies indicated, but these are among the most common.

- Nux vomica 30c

For competitive, ambitious workaholic, who becomes exhausted from overwork or overindulgence.

- Sepia 30c

For the worn-out, weepy woman. Feels distant from family. Depressed and dislikes company. Feels the cold easily. May be better for exercise.

DOSAGE 1 tablet twice daily. Maximum 5 days.

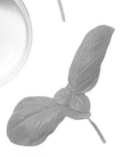

LEFT Basil oil is a good mental stimulant.

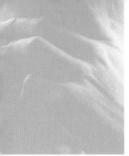

Chronic fatigue syndrome

Fatigue from a particular date onward; unexplained muscle weakness, often with painful joints or muscles, forgetfulness and difficulty in concentrating, mood swings, and depression.

While whole volumes have been written about chronic fatigue syndrome, there is still controversy about its nature, with some experts believing that it is wholly a psychological illness. Typified by grinding fatigue, an inability to stay awake, muscle pains, mood swings, and loss of concentration, enthusiasm and appetite—often leading to severe depression—chronic fatigue syndrome is hard to treat. The only route to long-term success is to combine medical treatment with self-help and the support of family and friends. Healthy eating is the basis of recovery, and extreme dietary regimes of any sort should be avoided.

 Call the physician

If symptoms of chronic fatigue syndrome persist.

 CONVENTIONAL MEDICINE

Because the cause of this illness is not known, there is no specific conventional remedy that has been shown to be more effective than any other. Most physicians recommend taking gentle, graded exercise, with rest periods when the symptoms are particularly severe. Eat a healthy diet. Take measures to limit stress, and consider undergoing counseling.

 HERBAL REMEDIES

Herbal immune stimulants, such as echinacea (avoid if you are pregnant or have a disorder of the immune system) and astragalus (avoid if pregnant), can help in the long term, while tonic herbs (such as damiana) provide an energy boost during recovery, but taking them too soon can exhaust the system.

USE AND DOSAGE Use drop doses of bitters, like wormwood or gentian tinctures, before meals to improve the digestion.

An infusion using equal amounts of vervain, betony, and oatstraw can help with depression.

A daily bowl of shiitake mushroom soup acts as an immune tonic and restorative.

Take 1g of evening primrose oil daily.

NUTRITION

Do not go more than 3 hours without eating, and eat natural-sugar foods like dried fruits when you need a boost. Take a daily high-dose multivitamin and mineral supplement.

Eat plenty of brown rice and whole wheat bread and pasta for their energy; liver, all the legumes and dark green vegetables for their B vitamins; citrus fruits, salads, and vegetables for their vitamin C. Avoid alcohol, all caffeine, sugar, sweets, candies, and any other foods that have a poor nutritional value.

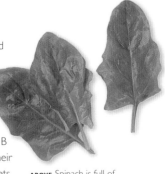

ABOVE Spinach is full of iron and chlorophyll, as well as B vitamins.

AROMATHERAPY

FOR MUSCULAR FATIGUE:
- Thyme *(Thymus vulgaris)*
- Lemon grass *(Cymbopogon citratus)*
- Marjoram *(Origanum majorana)*

FOR INSOMNIA *(SEE ALSO P.38)*:
- Valerian *(Valeriana fauriei)*
- Roman chamomile *(Chamaemelum nobile)*

FOR DEPRESSION:
- Neroli *(Citrus aurantium)*
- Rose *(Rosa centifolia/Rosa damascena)*

These oils are soothing, warming, and uplifting. Do not use marjoram on babies or small children. Avoid valerian if you have a skin injury or disorder or a heart condition.

APPLICATION Use in baths, foot spas, for massage, and in inhalations. Professional help from an aromatherapist can help see you through this problem.

Prevention

The general consensus is that chronic fatigue syndrome is caused by a viral infection, so the only preventative measure may be maintenance of an adequate and efficient immune system.

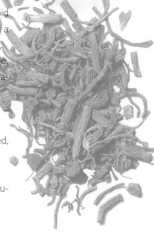

HOMEOPATHIC REMEDIES

There are many homeopathic remedies indicated, but these are among the most common.

- Carbolic acid 6c

For mental and physical fatigue. Belching and nausea. Band-like headaches. Craves stimulants.

- Calcarea carbonica 6c

For chilly, sweaty head, especially at night. Hardworking, takes on too much. Lots of sore throats.

DOSAGE I tablet daily. Maximum 2 weeks.

ABOVE Valerian makes a soothing oil for those with chronic fatigue.

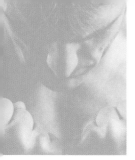

Stress

Typified by lots of minor medical ailments, often all at the same time, and possibly including a fast heartbeat; diarrhea; an edgy or depressed feeling; difficulty sleeping; poor or increased appetite; irritability.

I t is most important to realize that some stress is an essential ingredient of everyday life. What varies is the way in which people cope with different levels of stress. Once you have learned the levels you can comfortably withstand, it is not difficult to learn the skills needed to cope with higher stress levels. Whatever causes your stress, your body's response is the same. Large amounts of adrenalin are poured into your system, preparing you for "flight or fight." Difficulties arise when you cannot do either. In most cases counseling, psychotherapy, and relaxation techniques can help, but home remedies play a major part, too.

 Call the doctor

If you have been feeling consistently stressed for more than 2 weeks.

 CONVENTIONAL MEDICINE

Following a stressful episode, try to reorganize events to avoid further upset. Eat regular meals and take regular exercise—consider yoga or meditation relaxation therapy. Try to avoid resorting to alcohol or cigarettes. If the symptoms become unmanageable, your physician may be able to make a referral to a counselor. Drugs to control the symptoms or lift your mood are not a panacea, but may improve the symptoms to a point at which you are more able to help yourself.

 HERBAL REMEDIES

Relaxing herbs like betony, lemon balm, lavender, camomile, vervain, or skullcap make ideal teas to soothe tensions and nervous stress. Valerian is ideal for easing tensions: the taste is distinctive, so tablets may be preferable (avoid if you have a skin injury or disorder or a heart condition).

USE AND DOSAGE Use 1–2tsp of the relaxing herbs per cup of tea.

Siberian ginseng will help the body cope with stress: take 600mg daily in the week before expected stresses occur.

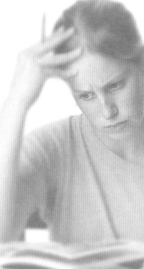

✿ HOMEOPATHIC REMEDIES

There are many remedies indicated, but these are among the most common. A consultation with a qualified homeopath is recommended.

☙ Nux vomica 30c

For a competitive, impatient, ambitious go-getter. Symptoms of abdominal pain, which is cramping. Likes coffee, spices, alcohol, and fats. Stress from overwork.

DOSAGE 1 tablet twice daily. Maximum 5 days.

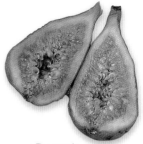

ABOVE Figs contain serotonin, which can calm the mind and body.

🍎 NUTRITION

It is hard to overemphasize the role of nutrition in helping to calm a stressful life. Serotonin and tryptophan both have a calming effect on mind and body. For serotonin, eat plenty of nuts (especially walnuts), dates, figs, pineapples, papayas (avoid if pregnant), passion fruit, tomatoes, avocados, and eggplant. For tryptophan, eat plenty of potatoes, beans, pasta, rice, and whole wheat bread. Get your protein from modest amounts of fish, poultry, and low-fat dairy products, as well as beans and cereals. The B vitamins and iron are also very important requirements for managing stress. Use herbs like thyme, lemon balm, basil (avoid if pregnant), lemon verbena, and nutmeg (avoid if allergic to nuts) in generous quantities for their calming effects. Avoid excessive consumption of mental irritants, such as alcohol and the caffeine in cola, coffee, tea, and chocolate.

COFFEE BEANS

> **Prevention**
> *Planning your life to minimize overcommitment and learning to say "no" are the first steps in prevention. Yoga, meditation, relaxation exercises, massage, and calming baths may all help.*

💧 AROMATHERAPY

The range of effective oils is vast, so pick ones whose aroma you like: perhaps lavender, geranium, patchouli, clary sage, or petitgrain; any of the citrus oils; the floral oils—niaouli, rose, jasmine (do not give to babies or small children), ylang ylang; woody oils such as cedarwood; vetivert. If your stress is a digestive, muscular, or menstrual problem, look under those ailments.

APPLICATION Do not make a complex regime that creates even more stress. Put the oil in the bath and just enjoy the pleasure of it.

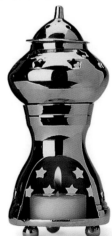

BELOW An aromatherapy burner is simple to use but yields huge benefits.

Insomnia

*Difficulty getting to sleep,
which may occur at any
time during normal
sleeping hours.*

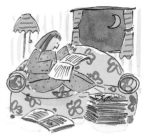

None of us can escape the occasional bad night's sleep. Real insomnia,
however, is a state of habitual sleepless-
ness, repeated night after night, often for months or even years on end.
Worrying about insomnia, to the point of obsession, does more damage
than the lack of sleep itself. But in most instances better sleep hygiene
and a wealth of home remedies can help you get the sleep of the just.

BELOW Taking exercise
during the day will help
you sleep at night.

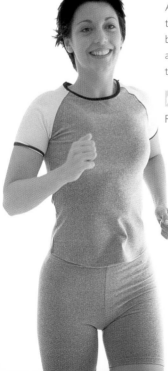

 CONVENTIONAL MEDICINE

Stop working at least an hour before bedtime.
Have a hot milky drink and a bath (but not too
hot). Avoid alcohol. Go to bed, but if you are awake
after 30 minutes, get up and settle into a relaxing
activity, such as reading a newspaper or magazine.
After 30 minutes go back to bed. Repeat as many
times as necessary. During the day (never just
before bedtime), perform regular aerobic exercise,
at least three times a week. Seek medical advice if
the symptoms of insomnia persist.

 HERBAL REMEDIES

Relaxing herbs to help ensure that you get a restful
night's sleep include valerian, hops, passion
flower, and skullcap.

USE AND DOSAGE These herbs are available as
tinctures or capsules.

Also worth trying is a combination of
passion flower, lavender, and betony—use
these herbs in equal amounts in an infusion
as a nighttime drink.

Cowslip flowers are a traditional and effective
remedy for insomnia associated with overexcite-
ment. Use a tincture and take 20–40 drops in
hot milk before bed.

NUTRITION

Going to bed too full or too hungry interferes with your normal sleep habits and thus leads to insomnia. Eating too late—especially a meal based on animal protein—is a great mistake, as such foods trigger greater production of the activity hormones. Evening meals should be based on starchy foods such as rice, pasta, potatoes, root vegetables, and beans, saving meat meals for the middle of the day.

ABOVE An evening meal centered on pasta will satisfy your hunger.

Eat plenty of fish, poultry, liver (in limited quantities or not at all if you're pregnant), eggs, potatoes, brown rice, whole grain cereals, whole wheat bread, and soy products, which are the best sources of vitamin B_6, lack of which can be a factor in insomnia. Culinary herbs can also be a tremendous help, especially sage and rosemary (avoid both if pregnant.)

AROMATHERAPY

- Lavender *(Lavandula angustifolia)*
- Clary sage *(Salvia sclarea)*
- Orange *(Citrus aurantium/Citrus sinensis)*
- Marjoram *(Origanum majorana)*
- Basil *(Ocimum basilicum)*

These oils are calming and soothing. Basil helps to clear the mind (avoid if you are pregnant); marjoram is a warming muscle-relaxant (do not use on babies or small children).

APPLICATION Use in a warm bath, or put a couple of drops on the pillow, in a burner in the bedroom.

HOMEOPATHIC REMEDIES

- Passiflora 30c

For restless, wakeful sleep. Try this remedy first.

- Nux vomica 30c

For overworked person, who wakes in early hours thinking of work. Wakes with hungover feeling.

- Coffea 30c

For waking in early hours, mind full of ideas, dreams disturb sleep. (Avoid if you have kidney disease, a heart condition, or an overactive thyroid.)

DOSAGE 1 tablet taken before bed for 10 days or until improved.

Caution

Avoid sleeping tablets, which are addictive. They may be suitable for short-term treatment under medical supervision. Never drink alcohol or drive if you are using clary sage oil. It has a powerful sedative effect and combines badly with alcohol.

Prevention

A regular sleep routine is vital and depends on going to bed and getting up at roughly the same time every day— insomnia is quite rare in those who have to be up at 6:00 A.M. Do not allow yourself to sleep during the day, as this will make getting back to normal even more difficult.

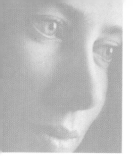

Seasonal affective disorder: SAD

BASIL

Characterized by mood changes related to the seasons; it is often associated with a craving for carbohydrates, lethargy, fatigue, and insomnia.

W hen the retina at the back of the eye is stimulated by light, the pineal gland in the brain decreases its production of the hormone melatonin, which helps regulate sleep cycles. During the winter months, when there is not much sunlight, more melatonin is released. Some people are much more severely affected by this lack of daylight than others and become extremely depressed and lethargic.

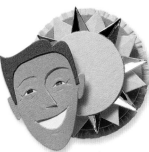

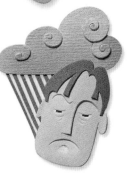

ABOVE Dramatic mood swings can make your life unbearable, but small lifestyle changes can make a big difference.

CONVENTIONAL MEDICINE

Light therapy—daily exposure to a light box or other bright light source—can help in many cases.

HERBAL REMEDIES

St. John's wort is an effective anti-depressant. For uplift, eat plenty of fresh basil and inhale the scent of the crushed leaves (avoid if pregnant).

USE AND DOSAGE Take 300mg of St. John's wort three times daily for 4 to 6 weeks.

Also try taking 600mg of Siberian ginseng daily for 4 to 6 weeks in early winter.

HOMEOPATHIC REMEDIES

This problem is complex to treat, so consult a qualified homeopath. The following remedies offer only a brief guide.

Sepia 30c

For person who cannot be bothered, even with family. Feels separated from them and depressed. Guilty feelings and tearful. Slow mentally and sharp-tongued. Better after exercise.

Aurum 30c

For depressed, sulky, weepy person. All emotions felt in the extreme. Critical of both self and others.

DOSAGE 1 tablet daily. Maximum 5 days.

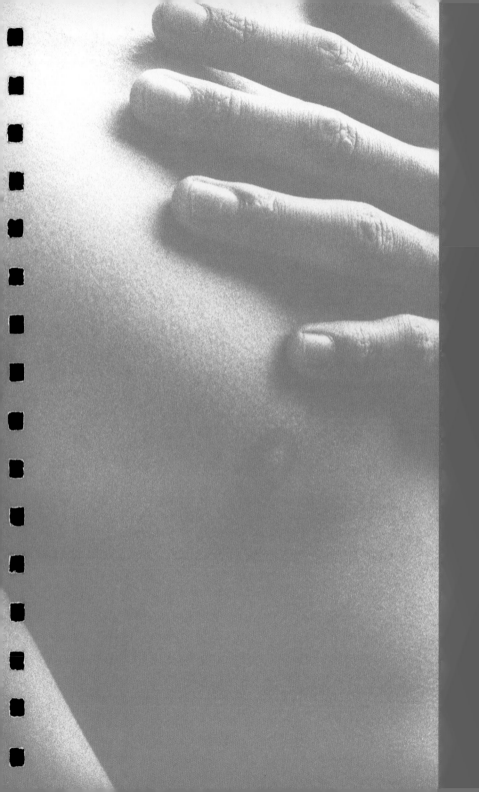

The
Respiratory
System

Every minute we take approximately 12 breaths, drawing oxygen into our lungs and expelling carbon dioxide, but since this generally occurs automatically, we often ignore the respiratory system until something goes wrong with it. Viruses, irritation of the mucous membranes, and inhaled pollutants can all threaten the respiratory tract, leading to coughs and colds, asthma, and hay fever. This section suggests easy remedies to make these common ailments more bearable.

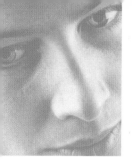

Congestion

Typified by excessive amounts of thick mucus in the nose, throat, and chest, which is caused by infection, allergy, or irritation of the mucous membranes; plus a blocked or runny nose.

Irritation of the mucous membranes in the nose and throat, or allergic reactions, can cause an increase in the amount of mucus produced by these tissues. Viral or bacterial infections can also produce the same reaction and, if the sinuses become congested and infected, the result can be sinusitis *(see p.50)*.

Prevention
Stop smoking and avoid exhaust fumes, chemical smells, and other irritant pollutants. Avoid allergens (see Allergies on p.14). Blow your nose often to reduce the risk of infection.

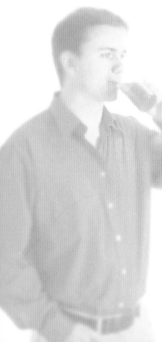

 CONVENTIONAL MEDICINE

Congestion will improve without treatment, usually within a week or two. However, steam inhalations *(see p.196)* make the mucus thinner and breathing more comfortable, and help to reduce the swelling; they can be used as often as necessary. Decongestants help too, particularly those that are sprayed up the nose. Beware: if continued for more than a week, a nasal decongestant will actually make the nose more stuffy than it was before.

DOSAGE: ADULTS AND CHILDREN Most nasal decongestants should be sprayed into the nose at least twice a day.

 HERBAL REMEDIES

A combination of astringent and soothing herbs will help clear congestion and ease inflammation.

USE AND DOSAGE Try mixing equal amounts of dried elderflower, eyebright, marshmallow leaves, and English plantain, then use in infusions (2tsp to a cup of boiling water, four times a day).

Steam inhalants can also help. Mix 5 drops each of sandalwood (avoid if you have a kidney problem), and eucalyptus oils with 1tsp of friar's balsam (compound tincture of benzoin) in a basin of boiling water and then inhale for 10 minutes. Do not use eucalyptus if you have digestive problems or liver disease; do not give to infants or small children.

AROMATHERAPY

- Eucalyptus *(Eucalyptus radiata)*
- Benzoin *(Styrax benzoin)*
- Thyme *(Thymus vulgaris)*

These oils relieve congestion and help to fight infection. But if congestion is due to an allergy *(see p.14)*, then lavender or chamomile oil may be more beneficial. Do not use eucalyptus if you have digestive problems or liver disease.

APPLICATION Steam inhalation and/or facial massage from a therapist are generally beneficial.

HOMEOPATHIC REMEDIES

There are many congestion remedies (see *also Sinusitis on p.50*). If the following do not help, then consult a homeopath.

- Kali bichromicum 6c

For thick, ropy, gluey, green or yellow phlegm. Pressing pain in root of nose. Dry crusts in nose. Worse for hot weather.

- Pulsatilla 6c

For stuffed-up nose, white/yellow-green discharge. Better in open air. Loss of smell or foul smell in nose from phlegm. Ears may discharge.

- Sambucus nigra 6c

For snuffles in babies, with difficulty suckling.

DOSAGE 1 tablet every 4 hours until condition improves. Maximum 12 doses.

NUTRITION

Naturopaths believe that a high consumption of dairy products can increase the production of mucus. So cut down on all milk-based foods for a couple of weeks. If you do this for any longer, get professional guidance about your diet and about supplements, to prevent calcium and other deficiencies.

Eat plenty of onions, chives, spring onions, leeks, and garlic, all traditional decongestants; sweet potatoes, carrots, broccoli, and red or dark green cabbage for their beta-carotene. Add thyme, ginger (avoid if you have gallstones), and chilis (avoid if pregnant) to recipes, as these are decongestants.

Caution

These oils (excluding the lavender and chamomile) are all very strong and should probably not be used for small children.

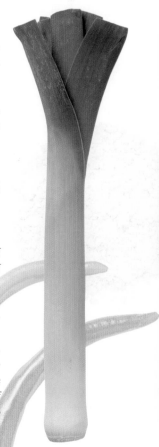

BELOW Leeks, chilis, and ginger can all bring relief from congestion.

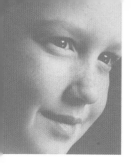

Common cold

Characterized by sneezing, runny nose, cough, congestion, and a sore, scratchy throat; often accompanied by generalized muscular aches and pains, together with a lack of energy and sometimes, a low-grade fever.

Hundreds of different viruses are responsible for the symptoms of a cold, and coughing or sneezing in confined spaces, and shaking hands with a cold sufferer, are effective ways of transmitting them. Having defied the combined efforts of the world's physicians, virologists, and other experts, the common cold is one condition for which the old wives' tales often produce the best results. So encourage your body's defenses by getting plenty of rest, eating a nutritious diet, and enjoying the benefits of steam treatment and other home remedies.

Caution
Always read pain reliever labels carefully, and make sure that you do not exceed the stated dose.

BELOW A cold may affect your sense of taste, but try to eat a balanced diet.

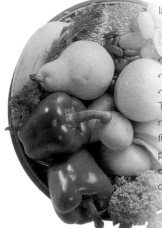

CONVENTIONAL MEDICINE

Fever and malaise can be treated with pain-relievers, which often need to be continued for several days until the symptoms subside. Inhalations of steam *(see p.196)* as often as possible help to make breathing easier. Babies may need nose drops to enable them to breathe more easily while feeding. Colds usually last between 3 and 10 days.

DOSAGE: ADULTS 1–2 tablets of pain relievers at onset, then every 4 hours; consult labels for details.

DOSAGE: CHILDREN Give regular doses of children's pain reliever (do not give aspirin to a child with a fever, due to its link with Reye's syndrome); consult label, or follow medical advice.

AROMATHERAPY

- Eucalyptus *(Eucalyptus radiata)*
- Tea tree *(Melaleuca alternifolia)*
- Pine *(Pinus sylvestris)*

Tea tree will make you sweat, which helps to eliminate the virus (make sure that you drink extra fluid). Do not use pine if you have a heart problem, problems breathing, or a skin injury. Do not use eucalyptus if you have digestive problems or liver disease; do not give to infants or small children.

APPLICATION Use these oils in vaporizers or inhalations to ease congestion. Or put them in the bath, using tea-tree oil at the first onset of symptoms.

❋ HOMEOPATHIC REMEDIES

Aconite 30c
For first signs of cold. Frequent sneezing, nose stuffed up. Thirsty, worse for stuffy rooms.

Allium cepa 30c
For profuse sneezing, streaming eyes and nose. Hot, thirsty, better in fresh air. Nose sore.

Natrum muriaticum 30c
For cold that begins with sneezing. Discharge from nose, like the white of an egg. Nose may also be blocked. Cold sores, mouth ulcers, and cracked lips.
DOSAGE I tablet up to every 4 hours, as needed. Maximum 3–4 days.

🍎 NUTRITION

Eat plenty of fresh fruit, salads, and raw vegetables; at least two cloves of raw garlic daily (onions and garlic have a powerful antiseptic and decongestant effect); thick onion soup or oven-baked onions daily. Drink plenty of fluids to replace those lost through sweating, but stick mainly to fruit juices, plain water, herbal teas, and a hot water, lemon, and honey mixture (not for children under two). Avoid dairy products and all sugary food for 2 or 3 days.

🌿 HERBAL REMEDIES

Herbs can ease many symptoms of a cold, and some display antiviral activity to combat the cause.
USE AND DOSAGE Tea made from equal parts of elder-flower, peppermint (use catmint instead for children—avoid if you have a gallbladder or liver problem), yarrow, and hyssop (I tsp per cup, taken up to four times daily) eases congestion, chills, and coughs.

Gargling with a standard infusion of sage will soothe sore throats (avoid if pregnant).

Take 200mg of echinacea up to 5 times a day for up to 4 days. (Avoid if you are pregnant or have a disorder of the immune system.)

Prevention
Eat plenty of pumpkin seeds, oysters, and other shellfish to keep your zinc intake up to the mark. When there are lots of colds around, suck 3 or 4 zinc and vitamin C lozenges each day to boost your immunity.

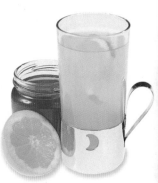

ABOVE A hot lemon and honey drink makes you feel better, as well as having nutritional benefits.

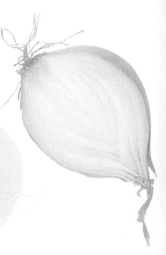

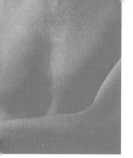

Coughs and bronchitis

The explosive release of air from the lungs, caused by inflammation of the bronchi, the larger air passages leading to the lungs; mucus that is clear or colored, often yellow or brown; a dry, scratchy throat.

cough may be due to nothing more than inhaled irritants like dust, exhaust fumes, smoke, or a crumb of food. Of all symptoms in the respiratory tract, a cough is the commonest, but it may be a sign of underlying illness. Acute bronchitis, however, is caused by an infection, often following flu or a severe cold. Chronic bronchitis, most common in cool, damp climates, is caused by repeated irritation from damp air and smoking, leading to an overproduction of mucus. This reduces the amount of oxygen available, making the heart work harder. A chest infection on top of chronic bronchitis causes severe breathing problems.

 Call the physician

If you have a deep cough; if you are coughing up bloodstained mucus, which may be a sign of more serious illness.

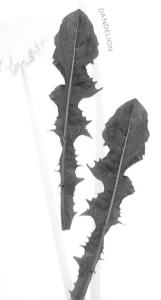

DANDELION

 CONVENTIONAL MEDICINE

A dry cough will often be relieved by a steam inhalation (see p.196), which you can have as often as necessary. If a cough does not clear up within 2–3 weeks, see your physician. A deeper cough, such as the type that develops after a cold into bacterial lung infection (most common in children and the elderly) may require antibiotics. There is no evidence that cough medicines have any effect.

 NUTRITION

For all respiratory problems a daily bowl of garlic soup is invaluable, as it is both decongestant and antibacterial. Eat plenty of celery, parsley (avoid if you are pregnant or have a heart or kidney condition), and fresh dandelion leaves (avoid if you have a bowel or gallbladder problem) to increase urinary output and help eliminate toxins; onions and leeks (the same family as garlic); fish, legumes, brown rice, and bananas for their B vitamins; liver, carrots, sweet potatoes, and spinach for their vitamin A; oily fish for their anti-inflammatory properties. Cut out all salt in order to prevent fluid retention. Reduce your intake of all dairy products to help lessen mucus formation.

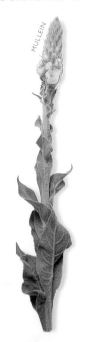

MULLEIN

HERBAL REMEDIES

Herbal cough remedies can ease bronchial spasms, expel phlegm, lubricate a dry cough or suppress an irritant one.

Use and Dosage For chesty coughs or bronchitis, use thyme, elecampane, mullein, cowslip, white horehound, or Iceland moss in teas (1tsp per cup) sweetened with honey (not for children under two).

A syrup can be made by layering slices of onion or turnip with sugar; leave overnight, then drink the liquid in 1tsp doses.

Cough suppressants like wild cherry can ease nervous, irritant coughs but should be avoided when trying to expel phlegm.

HOMEOPATHIC REMEDIES

Rumex 6c
For throat tickling with cold air, spasmodic dry cough preventing sleep. Hoarseness. Phlegm tough, worse for talking and cold air. Better for covering the mouth.

Bryonia 6c
For dry, hacking, spasmodic cough. Must sit up. Worse for eating, drinking, at night. Cough on entering warm room. Holds chest on coughing.

Dosage 1 tablet three times daily until improved. Maximum 2 weeks.

AROMATHERAPY

- Sandalwood *(Santalum album)*
- Benzoin *(Styrax benzoin)*
- Eucalyptus *(Eucalyptus radiata)*
- Frankincense *(Boswellia sacra)*
- Tea tree *(Melaleuca alternifolia)*

Steam inhalations are soothing. Throat massage eases tension. Gargling ensures that no infection sets in. Avoid eucalyptus if you have digestive problems or liver disease; do not give to infants or small children. Avoid sandalwood if you have a kidney problem.

Application Use sandalwood, benzoin, eucalyptus, or frankincense in steam inhalations. Massage the throat/chest with any of these; use tea tree for gargles.

Prevention

Don't smoke. Avoid other smokers. Keep the lungs in good condition through regular exercise. Keep bedrooms cool and well aired. Consider installing an air purifier. Wear a protective mask for all dusty do-it-yourself jobs and when air-pollution levels are high.

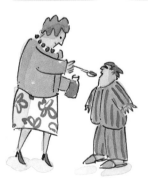

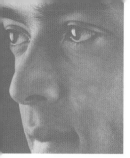

Hay fever

Typified by repeated sneezing fits; either a blocked or a constantly runny nose; sore, itchy eyes, which may be inflamed; a tickle in the roof of the mouth.

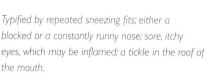

HONEY BEE

Hay fever is an allergic reaction to the pollen produced by grasses that mainly flower in the spring and summer. The sore, puffy eyes, runny nose, and violent bouts of sneezing are instantly recognizable. But it is not only grass pollens that cause hay fever—today the term is often used to describe allergic reactions to other airborne irritants, like exhaust fumes, general atmospheric pollution, and even strong smells, like some perfumes. Some unfortunate people suffer constantly from hay fever symptoms—a condition known as perennial rhinitis, most often caused by the droppings of the house dustmite.

✚ CONVENTIONAL MEDICINE

Drug treatments come as eyedrops, tablets, and nose sprays (do not use for more than 7 days).
DOSAGE: ADULTS Take most tablets once a day; eyedrops more often; consult label, or follow medical advice. Apply 2 puffs of spray per nostril twice a day.
DOSAGE: CHILDREN Doses of antihistamine syrup depend on the age of the child; consult label, or follow medical advice. For children over six, apply 2 puffs of nose spray per nostril twice a day.

❖ HOMEOPATHIC REMEDIES

Hay fever can be treated with mixed pollens (30c taken once every two weeks during the season). Homeopathic tablets can be bought over the counter; alternatively try one of the following:

 Allium cepa 6c
For running, sore nose, watering but not sore eyes. Worse for warm rooms. Better in the open air.

 Euphrasia 6c
For watery and sore eyes, running but not sore nose. Worse for light and warmth.
DOSAGE I tablet twice daily. Maximum 2 weeks.

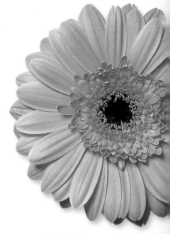

HERBAL REMEDIES

Herbalists often treat hay fever by using strengthening and cleansing herbs for the respiratory tract early on in the year, before the problem becomes too severe.

USE AND DOSAGE Make a tea out of comfrey and fenugreek and drink 1–2 cups of this infusion daily for several months before the onset of the hay fever season.

To relieve symptoms that occur during the actual hay fever season, take eyebright in capsules (up to 8 × 200mg daily) and bathe the eyes with either well-strained, sterilized marigold or eyebright infusions.

ABOVE Gently bathing the eyes in a flower infusion can bring relief from itchiness.

AROMATHERAPY

🌿 Roman chamomile *(Chamaemelum nobile)*

🌿 Basil *(Ocimum basilicum)*

🌿 Melissa *(Melissa officinalis)*

Chamomile and melissa are both anti-allergens; basil helps to clear the sinuses and the head of the nasty effects of hay fever (avoid if pregnant).

APPLICATION Place 1 drop of each oil on a handkerchief, which you can then carry with you for instant relief. You can also use these oils for massaging the upper back and chest.

NUTRITION

Reduce your intake of dairy products—naturopaths believe they increase mucus formation, which may exacerbate the problem. If this helps and you make permanent changes to your diet, make sure that you replace the missing nutrients (especially the calcium) from other sources. Vitamin C and its accompanying bioflavonoids are important protectors of the mucous membranes. All berries and fresh currants supply large quantities of both, and citrus fruits (including some of the pith and skin) should also be eaten in abundance.

If you have a pollen allergy, eating 4tsp daily of locally produced honey (not for children under two) can provide great relief.

Prevention

If you suffer from pollen allergy, stay indoors early in the morning and late in the evening, keep the windows closed, and wear wrap-around sunglasses.

BELOW Strawberries contain a surprising amount of vitamin C.

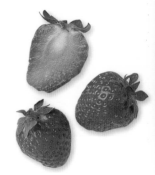

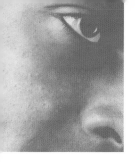

Sinusitis

*Pain in the face or gums, a persistent headache, often over
the eyes; pain worse on leaning forward; foul taste in the
mouth; bloodstained discharge from the nose; completely or
partially blocked nose.*

A heavy cold, allergies, irritant fumes, smoking, upper respiratory
infections, nasal polyps or adverse reactions to some foods may
all be the cause of sinusitis. This inflammation of the membranes lining
the sinuses, and their consequent overproduction of mucus, is what
produces the symptoms of headaches, facial pain, stuffiness, loss of
smell, pain in the teeth, repeated episodes of chest and ear infections,
and thick, infected mucus. While antibiotics may be essential to treat
severe infections, home remedies are best for milder conditions as well
as for prevention.

BELOW Home remedies
might need to be
supplemented by antibiotic
treatment for a severe or
prolonged attack of sinusitis.

 CONVENTIONAL MEDICINE

Treatment involves improving drainage from the
sinus, together with eliminating the infection. Steam
helps to make the mucus thinner and reduces nasal
congestion. Nose sprays containing decongestants
may help, but if used for too long can make the
congestion worse. Antibiotics may be needed to
clear the infection. Recurrent sinusitis may require
surgical treatment.

 HERBAL REMEDIES

Decongestant herbs. such as chamomile, elderflower, coltsfoot (avoid if pregnant), yarrow,
eyebright, or plantain, are all beneficial.

USE AND DOSAGE Make teas using 2tsp of herb per
cup: add a pinch of goldenseal (avoid if pregnant) or
bayberry powder or 5 drops of tincture, if available.

Gently massaging the sinus areas with a cream or
infused oil containing any of these herbs will help.

Add 10 drops each of peppermint (avoid if you
have a gallbladder or liver problem), pine (avoid if
you have a heart problem, problems breathing, or
a skin injury), and sandalwood (avoid if you have a
kidney problem) oils to a basin of hot water and
inhale for up to 10 minutes.

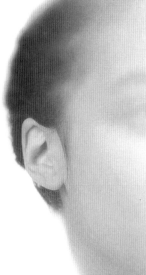

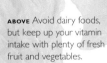

✿ HOMEOPATHIC REMEDIES

There are many remedies that help sinusitis. If these
do not help, consult a qualified homeopath.

 Kali bichromicum 6c

For thick, yellow, ropy phlegm. Pulsating pain
at root of nose and frontal sinuses worse
for stooping. Pressure in ear. Worse for
drafts and cold, dry weather. Loss of smell.

Hepar sulphuris calcareum 6c

For thick, white or yellow, smelly phlegm that
makes nose sore. Person irritable. Facial bones sore.
Right-sided shooting pains.

DOSAGE 1 tablet three times daily until improved.
Maximum 10 days.

ABOVE Avoid dairy foods,
but keep up your vitamin
intake with plenty of fresh
fruit and vegetables.

🍎 NUTRITION

The food that most commonly increases the production of mucus, especially in children, is cow's
milk, so try excluding cow's milk and milk products
from your diet for a few weeks. If this does help and
you are going to exclude them in the long term,
make sure you get plenty of calcium and vitamin D
from other sources (see Osteoporosis on p.70).

To maintain healthy sinuses, vitamins A, C, and E
and bioflavonoids are important, so eat plenty of
carrots, apricots, and dark green leafy vegetables;
citrus fruits, with some of the pith and skin; dark
cherries, tomatoes, and mangoes; avocados, olive,
sunflower, and safflower oils. Garlic, onions, and
leeks are all powerful weapons, while pineapple
juice is healing: drink at least three glasses, diluted
50:50 with water, each day. Reduce your salt intake
and go easy on the alcohol.

Prevention

*For those who are susceptible
to sinus problems, a monthly
2-day cleansing regime of
nothing but raw fruit,
vegetables, and salads—as
much as you like—with plenty
of fruit and vegetable juices
is highly beneficial.*

💧 AROMATHERAPY

Basil *(Ocimum basilicum)*
Tea tree *(Melaleuca alternifolia)*

These help to fight infection and clear the sinuses.
(Avoid basil if you are pregnant.)

APPLICATION Put the oils on a handkerchief, in a
burner, an electric vaporizer, a light ring, or just
a bowl of warm water. Steam inhalation is also effective for clearing the sinuses.

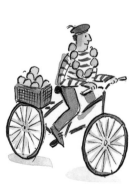

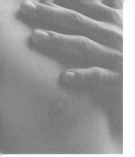

Asthma

Recurrent bouts of difficult breathing; tightness in the chest, usually associated with a wheezing cough, particularly at night (this cough may be the only apparent symptom in some children with asthma).

sthma is an extremely serious, potentially life-threatening illness. Attacks can be triggered by a wide variety of allergens and irritants, such as dust, pollen, animal dander, certain foods and drugs, air pollution, exercise, stress, even cold air. While the incidence of asthma is on the rise, particularly among children, a wide range of drug treatments as well as self-monitoring techniques are available to help control the disease. The following home remedies can improve your quality of life and reduce the frequency and severity of asthma attacks, but they are not meant to replace medical treatment or vigilant self-monitoring.

 Call the physician

If you are already asthmatic but have noticed recently that you need more medication than usual; if there is a rapid deterioration in your condition.

Caution

Avoid non-steroidal anti-inflammatory drugs, such as ibuprofen or aspirin, which may make your asthma worse.

 CONVENTIONAL MEDICINE

The goal of treatment is to prevent attacks by monitoring breathing capacity and taking inhaled drugs. Identifying and avoiding triggers is also key. See a doctor right away if you have a first-time attack.

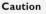 **HERBAL REMEDIES**

Herbal antispasmodics and broncho-dilators are very effective in treating asthma—although the most potent herbs, such as ephedra, are confined to professional use.

USE AND DOSAGE For mild cases, a steam inhalant of chamomile flowers (1tbsp to a basin of boiling water) can often avert an attack.

Macerate 2tsp of elecampane root overnight in a cup of cold water, then heat to boiling point; strain and sweeten with 1tsp of honey, then sip the liquid as required (not for children under two).

 HOMEOPATHIC REMEDIES

Asthma is a serious condition and may require medical attention. Do not stop taking medication prescribed by your physician. It helps to consult a qualified homeopath for this ailment.

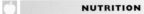

∽ Arsenicum album 6c

For wheezing, anxiety, restlessness, fear of suffocation. Worse 1:00–3:00 A.M., in cold air. Better for bending forward, warm drinks.

∽ Ipecacuanha 6c

For rattly chest, unable to cough up phlegm. Wheezy, chest feels tight. Cough with each breath. Nausea. Better for sitting up and in open air.

Dosage 1 tablet three times daily. Maximum period 1 week.

NUTRITION

In some cases of asthma, food and food additives can trigger attacks. Keep a detailed food diary, noting when attacks occur. This should give you some clues as to the foods that you would do well to avoid. Food additives, such as colorings, flavorings, and preservatives, can be severe triggers. Because dairy foods tend to increase the body's production of mucus, they can cause asthma problems. You may need professional guidance to make sure that you or your child does not suffer nutritional deficiencies if you start excluding major foods from the diet.

A diet that is rich in all the protective antioxidants that are so important for the health of lung tissue is essential. Salads, grapes, melons, tomatoes, bell peppers, kiwis, whole grain cereals, and lots of all the green vegetables should be the basis of the asthmatic's diet. Also drink plenty of water in order to keep hydrated and to loosen mucous secretions.

ABOVE Eat plenty of salads for a diet rich in antioxidants.

Caution

Do not use frankincense in a steam inhalation, as the heat will increase the inflammation of the mucous membrane, making the congestion worse.

AROMATHERAPY

∽ Frankincense *(Boswellia sacra)*

Frankincense slows and deepens breathing—it is used by monks when they are going into deep meditation. If asthma is an allergic reaction, try chamomile instead *(see also Stress on p.36)*.

Application Use in a vaporizer, compress, or bath, or for localized massage around the chest/facial area. Frankincense can also be put on a tissue or pillow to help you breathe.

BELOW If you find dairy products make asthma attacks worse or more frequent, eliminate them from your diet.

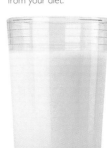

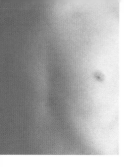

Hiccups

A sudden intake of breath, which is associated with a characteristic sound and sensation caused by a spasm of the diaphragm; often repeated several times before an episode stops.

I t is a sudden spasm of the diaphragm that causes a hiccup, triggered by irritation of the major nerve that supplies this muscle. Hiccups usually come in clusters and may last anywhere from a minute or so to hours, or even months. Attacks are nearly always the result of indigestion, overeating, rushing a meal, or consuming lots of carbonated drinks, although occasionally they may be a sign of an underlying and serious disease, such as liver abscess or kidney failure. Surprisingly, even medical textbooks suggest the traditional remedies of the cold key down the back or drinking from the wrong side of a glass.

BELOW Lie on your back with your knees bent.

BELOW Bring up your knees and pull them toward your chest as hard as you can.

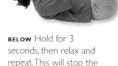

BELOW Hold for 3 seconds, then relax and repeat. This will stop the spasms that cause hiccups.

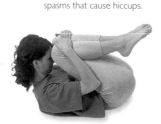

CONVENTIONAL MEDICINE

If hiccups persist, consult your physician, who may prescribe a drug to relax the diaphragm.

HOMEOPATHIC REMEDIES

🐍 Cajup 6c

For sudden attacks of hiccups at any provocation—talking, laughing, eating, or motion.

🐍 Ignatia 6c

For hiccups from emotional causes, when eating, drinking, or smoking. Empty sensation in stomach.

🐍 Cyclamen 6c

For hiccup-like belching. Worse for fatty food. Hiccups during pregnancy or while yawning.

🐍 Nux vomica 6c

For hiccups from overeating or -drinking.

DOSAGE 1 tablet every 30 minutes until improved. Maximum 12 doses.

HERBAL REMEDIES

USE AND DOSAGE Sip peppermint (avoid if you have a gallbladder or liver problem) or fennel infusion (avoid fennel if pregnant). Eat papaya fruit or juice (avoid if pregnant), or chew candied ginger (avoid if you have gallstones) or charcoal tablets.

The Circulatory System

Blood is pumped throughout the body by the heart at a rate of about 10pt/5liter per minute, but if for any reason this blood flow is restricted, then circulatory problems—for instance, varicose veins, chilblains, and restless legs—may result. If the blood's ability to absorb oxygen and convey it around the body is impaired, anemia may result. In both cases, home remedies, combined with regular exercise to stimulate the cardiovascular system, can make a major difference. Circulatory problems are, however, easier to prevent than to cure.

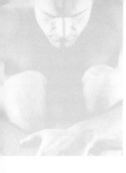

Anemia

*Characterized by tiredness; pale skin; shortness of breath
on even mild exertion; rapid heart rate and palpitations;
swollen ankles; a feeling of faintness and generalized
symptoms of fatigue.*

nemia is a condition in which the blood has a reduced ability to
absorb oxygen and transport it around the body in the form of
hemoglobin. Around 90 percent of all cases are the result of iron deficiency, usually caused by heavy or prolonged periods or by blood loss
from ulcers, hemorrhoids, or gum disease. Many women of childbearing
age are iron-deficient, while poor diet, deficiencies of folic acid and vitamin B$_{12}$, leukemia, sickle cell anemia, and thalassemia cause a few relatively rare cases. Vegetarians and pregnant women are vulnerable to
anemia. Dietary improvement is nearly always the answer.

 Call the physician

*If you think you are
suffering from anemia.*

 CONVENTIONAL MEDICINE

Because there are several different types of anemia,
you should consult your physician before taking any
treatment. Often a course of iron tablets is all that
is required, but some kinds of anemia do not need
any treatment, and iron may even make the condition worse. Your physician may have to order a
blood test in order to diagnose your condition.
Pregnant women often need to take iron and folic
acid supplements.

DOSAGE: ADULTS AND CHILDREN If you have iron deficiency, start with 1 iron tablet a day; see label for
details. Be aware that iron may cause constipation.

 NUTRITION

Always eat vitamin C-rich foods together with those
containing iron, in order to improve absorption.
Nettle soup and dandelion leaves (avoid dandelion if
you have a bowel or gallbladder problem) added to
salads are unusual but effective ways of getting lots
of extra iron. Add parsley (avoid if you are pregnant
or have a heart or kidney condition), chives, fennel
(avoid if you are pregnant), watercress, and elderber-
ries to salads and also to fruit dishes.

Eat plenty of organ meat for its vitamin B_{12}; meat, green vegetables, watercress, legumes, whole grain cereals, molasses, dried fruits, cashew nuts, wheatgerm, tomato paste, yeast extracts, and brewer's yeast for their iron and folic acid. For vegetarians a traditional vegetable curry cooked in a cast-iron container is an excellent source of iron that is well absorbed. In severe cases of anemia, food sources are not sufficient and supplements will form an essential part of your recovery.

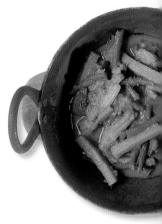

ABOVE Curry cooked in a cast-iron container has lots of easily absorbed iron.

 HERBAL REMEDIES

Stinging nettles and parsley (avoid both if pregnant or you have a heart or kidney condition) are rich in iron.
USE AND DOSAGE Make a tonic by steeping 3 cups/3½oz/100g each of stinging nettle, Chinese angelica /Dong Quai (avoid if pregnant), and dandelion root (avoid if you have a bowel or gallbladder problem) in 2pt/1 liter of red wine for 2 weeks; strain and drink one sherry glass per day.

Echinacea (2 × 200mg capsules daily) can help stimulate red blood-cell production. (Avoid if you are pregnant or have a disorder of the immune system.)

HOMEOPATHIC REMEDIES

The cause of anemia should be established first. A consultation with a qualified homeopath, who may work in conjunction with your physician, is suggested.

Ferrum metallicum 6c
For person who appears strong, flushed, has cold hands and feet, but feels weak after any effort. Hammering headache. Flushes easily from pain or emotions. Ringing in the ears before periods. Anemia due to heavy periods.

Calcarea phosphorica 6c
For children who are growing rapidly. Anemia after illness. Person dissatisfied with life and looking for something new. Tends to irritation.

China 6c
For anemia from blood loss. Feels weak, sensitive and nervous. Easily upset and feels chilly.
DOSAGE 1 tablet twice daily. Maximum 2 weeks.

> ## Prevention
> *Eat well and regularly, including all the foods listed under Nutrition. Avoid restrictive weight-loss diets or any other nutritional regime that seems extreme.*

BELOW Parsley and wine both contain iron.

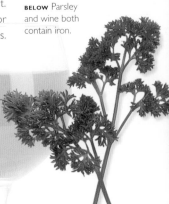

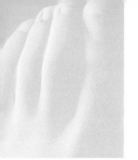

Chilblains/Frostbite

Painful, itchy, dark red swellings, which often affect the skin on the surface of the fingers and toes, but can also affect the ears, cheeks, and nose; if serious, chilblains may begin to ulcerate.

hese sore, itching, inflamed, and frequently swollen patches of skin occur most commonly on the backs of the fingers or tops of the toes. Sometimes they crop up on the ears, outer thighs, and other parts of the body that are subject to cold and/or pressure. The cause is restriction of the circulating blood supply in the capillaries—the tiniest blood vessels at the very end of the system—leading to lack of oxygen and nutrients, and consequent cell damage. Prevention is the only cure.

 Call the physician

If a chilblain begins to ulcerate.

 CONVENTIONAL MEDICINE

Avoid chilblains by wrapping up warmly in cold weather. Several thinner layers can be more effective than one thick one. Once developed, a chilblain may take several weeks to heal. Take pain relievers if required.

DOSAGE: ADULTS 1–2 tablets of pain relievers at onset of pain, repeated every 4 hours; see label for details.

DOSAGE: CHILDREN Give regular doses of children's pain reliever; consult label, or follow medical advice.

 HERBAL REMEDIES

Circulation can be improved with teas containing ginger (avoid if you have gallstones), cinnamon twigs (avoid if pregnant) or angelica root.

USE AND DOSAGE Simmer 1tsp of dried herb—either singly or in combination—with 2 cups of water for 10 minutes; add a pinch of cayenne powder before drinking (avoid cayenne if pregnant).

Cayenne cream can ease discomfort (may cause a burning sensation, do not use on broken skin), or try compresses containing oak-bark decoction.

Topical itching can be eased with arnica (do not use this, however, if the skin is broken and do not use internally) or marigold creams.

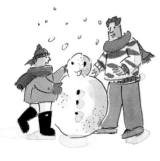

NUTRITION

Increase your consumption of vitamin E by eating plenty of avocados, all nuts and seeds, and olive oil; buckwheat (added to bread, cake, or cookie recipes, or as pancakes) for its rutin content; citrus fruits, blackcurrants, cherries, and blueberries for their vitamin C and bioflavonoids, which are essential nutrients for effective peripheral circulation. To prevent chilblains, take a daily dose of 400 IU of vitamin E and 1g of vitamin C with bioflavonoids. Also take a B-complex that includes nicotinic acid.

One unit of alcohol per day for women (two for men) will help open up the tiniest blood vessels. But larger amounts have the opposite effect, making chilblains worse. Caffeine in any form is a vasoconstrictor and reduces blood supply, as does nicotine.

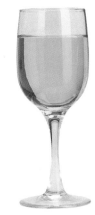

ABOVE A glass of white wine a day might open up tiny blood vessels and ease chilblains.

AROMATHERAPY

- Geranium *(Pelargonium graveolens)*
- Black pepper *(Piper nigrum)*
- Lavender *(Lavandula angustifolia)*

These oils are warming, soothing, increase the circulation, and have a slight painkilling effect.

APPLICATION Rub the oils, blended with either a carrier oil or a lotion, vigorously into the chilblains (but only unbroken ones). In the long term you should be looking at improving your circulation, either by massaging your feet or by using oils in the bath or in a foot bath. You could also use rosemary, lemon grass, or marjoram (not for babies or small children).

Caution
Anybody who is pregnant, suffering from high blood pressure or epilepsy should avoid rosemary oil.

HOMEOPATHIC REMEDIES

Calendula cream is often soothing for chilblains.

- Agaricus 6c

For burning, itching, and redness that is worse for cold.

- Petroleum 6c

For burning chilblains that itch, skin cracks.

- Plantago 6c

For skin that itches, burns, and is sensitive.

DOSAGE 1 tablet three times daily. Maximum 2 weeks.

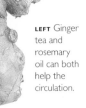

LEFT Ginger tea and rosemary oil can both help the circulation.

Varicose veins

Visible, often raised, unsightly, and painful distended veins that commonly appear in the legs, although they can also occur in the walls of the rectum (see Hemorrhoids on p.116); they may ache after standing for long periods.

aricose veins occur when valves in the veins fail to work properly and allow blood to flow backward or stagnate in the veins, causing them to bulge. There are often no symptoms, apart from an unsightly appearance. Although varicose veins are usually hereditary, they are often made worse by pregnancy, constipation, obesity, jobs that involve prolonged standing, and a sedentary lifestyle. If left untreated, varicose veins can cause swollen ankles, varicose eczema (scaling and itching of the skin above the affected veins), and in severe cases, ulcers or leg sores.

 Call the physician

If the skin starts to ulcerate over or near a varicose vein.

 CONVENTIONAL MEDICINE

Wearing special support stockings, walking regularly, losing weight, elevating the legs, and avoiding tight clothes and prolonged standing all help improve circulation. Varicose veins can be removed surgically.

 HOMEOPATHIC REMEDIES

⟳ Hamamelis 6c
For varicose veins that feel bruised and sore. Veins large, blue. Varicose veins in pregnancy.

⟳ Pulsatilla 6c
For legs that feel heavy. Varicose veins itchy in warmth.

⟳ Fluoricum acidum 6c
For painful varicose veins. Varicose ulcers that have red edges.

⟳ Ferrum metallicum 6c
For varicose veins during pregnancy.

DOSAGE 1 tablet twice daily until improved, or for 10 days. May be repeated.

 HERBAL REMEDIES

Buckwheat, which is rich in rutin, helps strengthen veins, while herbs such as sweet clover (avoid if pregnant), horse chestnut, witch hazel, motherwort, or yarrow can be used to improve circulation, combat any tendency to thrombosis, and counter the deposit of fibrin that can cause further damage. **USE AND DOSAGE** These herbs can be taken in teas or tinctures (try equal amounts of sweet clover, motherwort, or yarrow, for example).

Externally, distilled witch hazel or horse chestnut ointment can be used in gentle massage.

AROMATHERAPY

* Cypress *(Cupressus sempervirens)*
* Geranium *(Pelargonium graveolens)*

These oils are not only stimulating, they also help to increase circulation. (Avoid cypress if pregnant.)
APPLICATION Mix the essential oils with a carrier oil or lotion that can be massaged above the varicose veins—never over or below the veins. Place a warm compress on the vein if it is very painful and throbbing. Elevating your legs higher than your head for at least 10 minutes twice a day will also help. Avoid constipation (see p.96), as this simply puts even more pressure on the veins.

NUTRITION

If you already have varicose veins, make dietary changes to improve your intake of nutrients that are beneficial for circulation. Eat buckwheat—as pancakes, or added to bread or cookie recipes, for its rutin, a bioflavonoid that specifically strengthens blood vessels. Also eat plenty of avocados, olive oil, and all the nuts and seeds for their vitamin E; liver, sardines, eggs, shellfish, and pumpkin seeds for their zinc; and citrus fruits, blackcurrants, blackberries, blueberries, bilberries, and dark red cherries for bioflavonoids and vitamin C.

Excessive amounts of caffeine and alcohol have an adverse effect on the heart and blood vessels, thus reducing the efficiency of the circulatory system. A high salt intake encourages fluid retention, swelling, and high blood pressure, while refined carbohydrates and too much sugar lead to constipation and weight gain.

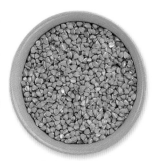
ABOVE Buckwheat helps strengthen veins so that blood won't pool in them.

Prevention
The main preventative step is to avoid constipation (see p.96)—plenty of fluids and the right kind of fiber are the key. And make lifestyle changes to control your weight.

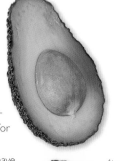
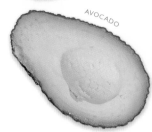
AVOCADO

Restless legs

PASSION FLOWER

Characterized by a burning feeling, weakness, or numbness, or by jerky movements in the legs, commonly occurring in women either just before going to sleep or soon after they sit down.

Symptoms of this usually minor, but nonetheless unpleasant, problem start as soon as you sit down or go to bed. Restless legs may be caused by prescribed drugs or by a problem in the central nervous system, but both these causes are unusual. More often, restless legs are a symptom of iron-deficiency anemia or are caused by circulation problems, and sometimes there is no apparent cause at all.

 Call the physician

If you suddenly start suffering from this problem and the condition is severe and intractable.

BELOW Boosting your iron intake might calm jerky legs that keep you awake at night.

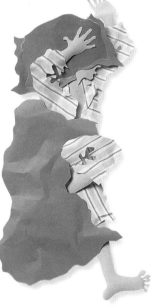

 CONVENTIONAL MEDICINE

Restless legs may occasionally be due to an iron deficiency, which can be easily treated by means of iron supplements.

HOMEOPATHIC REMEDIES

⁂ Zincum 6c

For twitching, constant movement of feet both night and day.

⁂ Tarantula 6c

For restless feet and legs in bed, with weakness and numbness. Restless sleep. Legs restless in evening and before going to bed.

DOSAGE 1 tablet three times daily. Maximum 2 weeks or until improved.

 HERBAL REMEDIES

Teas to soothe and relax the nerves are worth trying, especially chamomile, lemon balm, skullcap, vervain, and passion flower. If the problem is particularly severe at night, it is worth bathing the legs in cramp-bark decoction or massaging a little cream containing the herb into the legs before going to bed.

USE AND DOSAGE 1–2 drops of chamomile, rose, or lavender oil in 1tsp of almond oil also makes a good massage medium.

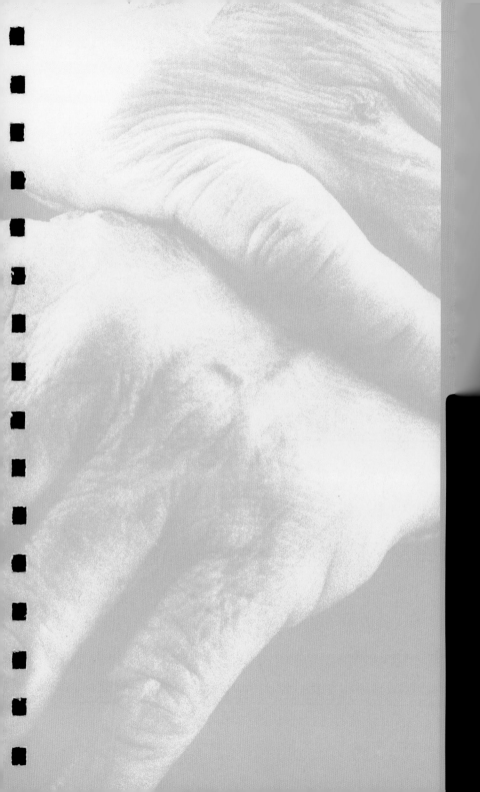

Bones and Muscles

The human skeleton contains more than 200 bones, which are moved by muscles and connected by ligaments and joints, giving us our complex body framework. Injuries, strains, wear and tear, and internal ill health can all affect this support system, causing aches and pains as well as more serious conditions. Today disorders of the musculoskeletal system make up 25 percent of all visits to the physician. This section looks at how such ailments—back pain or arthritis, osteoporosis or RSI—can be treated at home, so that we function at our optimum level.

Back pain

Pain may come on suddenly and resolve itself quickly, or it may become chronic and debilitating; often worse after sitting or standing for long periods; may affect any part of the spine; low back pain may be associated with pain down the leg.

ou have an almost 90 percent chance of suffering from back pain at some time in your life, and are then twice as likely to suffer again. Most back pain can be relieved by manipulative therapy within the first 6 weeks, though in some cases surgery may be the only answer. Prevention is the best treatment; if you are already a sufferer, try to maintain your back in a strong, healthy, and mobile state. Do not stay in bed for more than 48 hours, even with a severe attack—seek professional help as soon as possible.

 Call the physician

If you lose bowel or bladder control; if you suspect the pain is related to your kidneys; if you have numbness in a limb or difficulty moving it; if you experience pain passing down your leg; if you cannot control the pain; if there is no improvement after 4–6 weeks.

Caution

Make sure that back pain is properly diagnosed. Always read pain reliever labels carefully, and do not exceed the stated dose.

 CONVENTIONAL MEDICINE

Take a pain reliever regularly. This may need to be combined with a prescribed muscle relaxant. Try to avoid prolonged bed rest. If problems persist for more than a few days, early referral to a physiotherapist is recommended.

DOSAGE: ADULTS 1–2 tablets of pain relievers at onset of pain, repeated every 4 hours; consult label.

DOSAGE: CHILDREN Give regular doses of children's pain reliever; consult label, or follow medical advice.

 HERBAL REMEDIES

Herbal remedies can ease symptoms, but when back pain is related to a mechanical fault, like a slipped disk, manipulative treatment is preferable.

USE AND DOSAGE Castor oil packs (compresses that are soaked with warm castor oil) offer relief from back pain.

To ease local discomfort, soak a compress in ½ cup/100ml of hot water which contains crampbark (1tbsp) and cinnamon (1tsp) tinctures (avoid if pregnant), then apply to the affected area. Reheat and reapply as required. Anti-inflammatories such as devil's claw (avoid if you have an ulcer) (6 × 200mg capsules daily) can help.

NUTRITION

Eat plenty of celery and parsley (avoid if pregnant or if you have a heart or kidney condition) to encourage fluid elimination; turnips for their anti-inflammatory action; pineapple for its pain-relieving enzymes; and oily fish to maintain mobility. Reduce caffeine intake. Avoid carrying excessive weight.

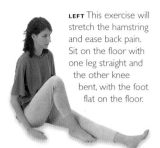

LEFT This exercise will stretch the hamstring and ease back pain. Sit on the floor with one leg straight and the other knee bent, with the foot flat on the floor.

 HOMEOPATHIC REMEDIES

Back pain associated with numbness or loss of bowel or bladder control requires immediate medical attention.

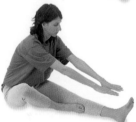

LEFT Allow the raised knee to fall to the side.

 Bryonia 6c

For stiffness in small of back at change of weather. Slow onset, worse for movement. Better for pressure, rest, and cold applications.

 Gnaphalium 6c

For pain extending down the leg, "sciatica" with numbness. Worse on right side, for lying down, and motion. Better for sitting in chair, drawing legs up.

 Tellurium 6c

For pain extending down the leg, sciatica, right-sided. Pain worse for cough, sneezing, opening the bowels, or touch. Also lumbago.

DOSAGE 1 tablet every 2–4 hours, for up to 3–4 days.

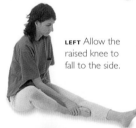

ABOVE Gently stretch your arms forward. Relax, then stretch again in a gentle rhythm for about 20 seconds. Repeat on the other side.

 AROMATHERAPY

Determining the cause of back pain is critical.

FOR MUSCULAR PROBLEMS:

 Lavender *(Lavandula angustifolia)*

 Marjoram *(Origanum majorana)*

FOR DISK PROBLEMS:

 Lavender *(Lavandula angustifolia)*

 Roman chamomile *(Chamaemelum nobile)*

 Marjoram *(Origanum majorana)*

The oils for muscular problems are warming and soothing; those for disk problems are soothing and help to kill the pain. Do not use marjoram for babies or small children.

APPLICATION Use the oils for muscular pain in a massage; use any of the recommended oils in the bath or in a compress.

BELOW Eat turnips as a natural alternative to prescribed anti-inflammatory drugs.

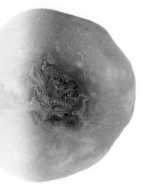

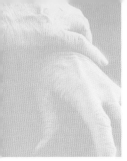

Arthritis

Aching, stiff joints, commonly in the fingers, wrists, elbows, shoulders, knees, ankles, and feet; joints are often swollen and sometimes deformed; symptoms may be minor or cause considerable pain.

There are more than 200 forms of arthritis that cause problems with the joints. Pain, stiffness, swelling, and inflammation are generally present, but conditions may range from the inconvenience of arthritis in a finger, caused by an injury 20 years before, to severe impairment from rheumatoid arthritis. Some of the more serious conditions do not lend themselves to home remedies, but whatever form of arthritis you have, diet can play a key role in reducing its severity. Osteoarthritis and rheumatoid arthritis also respond to self-help, though this is not a substitute for surgery or drug therapy.

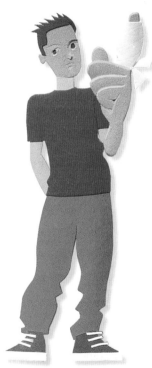

ABOVE Arthritis pain in the joints can be alleviated in part by changes in diet.

CONVENTIONAL MEDICINE

Relieve arthritis with simple pain relievers such as acetaminophen or aspirin. Sore joints may feel better when supported with a firm bandage. Keeping your joints warm may help, too, while gentle exercise is important to keep them supple.

DOSAGE: ADULTS 1–2 tablets of pain relievers at onset of pain, repeated every 4 hours; consult label for details.

DOSAGE: CHILDREN See a physician immediately if you suspect that a child has arthritis.

HERBAL REMEDIES

Anti-inflammatory herbs such as birch, black cohosh (avoid if pregnant), meadowsweet (do not take if you are sensitive to aspirin), and willow, are widely used—usually as teas, although birch sap was once a popular folk remedy. Devil's claw root is now popular (avoid if you have an ulcer).

USE AND DOSAGE Take up to 3g of devil's claw root powder daily in capsules, for at least 4 weeks.

Combine 10 drops of rosemary or wintergreen oil with 1tsp of infused comfrey oil (avoid comfrey and rosemary if pregnant), then use as a massage.

❖ HOMEOPATHIC REMEDIES

It is helpful to consult a qualified homeopath.

☞ **Bryonia 6c**

For joints that are red, hot, with tearing pains. Worse for slightest movement. Better for holding joint tightly, applying heat. Dry mouth and thirst.

☞ **Rhododendrum 6c**

For arthritis that affects smaller joints, which feel weak. Worse for changes of weather, and before storms and cold winters. Better for warmth.

DOSAGE 1 tablet three times daily. Maximum 1 month.

💧 AROMATHERAPY

☞ **Lavender** (*Lavandula angustifolia*)
☞ **Roman chamomile** (*Chamaemelum nobile*)
☞ **Eucalyptus** (*Eucalyptus radiata*)
☞ **Juniper** (*Juniperus communis*)
☞ **Ginger** (*Zingiber officinale*)

These oils have a painkilling effect. Avoid juniper if pregnant or if you have a kidney problem. Do not use eucalyptus if you have digestive problems or liver disease; do not give to infants or small children. Avoid ginger if you have gallstones.

APPLICATION Use in foot or hand baths, depending on where the affected joints are, or massage an oil or lotion into the body.

🍎 NUTRITION

Drink ginger tea and add plenty of ginger to recipes (avoid if you have gallstones). Include parsley (avoid if pregnant or if you have a heart or kidney condition), celery and watercress in your diet.

For all arthritic conditions, except gout, eat plenty of oily fish, for their omega-3 fatty acids; broccoli, carrots, and liver for their vitamin A and beta-carotene; citrus fruits, strawberries, and dark green vegetables for their vitamin C and bioflavonoids; olive oil, sunflower seeds, and avocados for their vitamin E. Reduce your intake of red meat, coffee, and game. Gout sufferers should reduce their alcohol intake and avoid game, organ meat, yeast and meat extracts, oily fish, fish roe, mussels, and scallops.

Prevention

Being seriously overweight adds greatly to the stresses on all weight-bearing joints and will predispose you to arthritis in the lower spine, hips, knees, ankles, and feet.

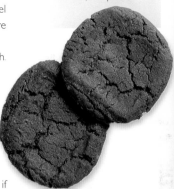

ABOVE Introduce ginger into your diet—in foods and in teas—and use it in oil for massage.

Caution

If you are using a compress, or a warm hand or foot bath (or just a warm bath), make sure that you mobilize the joints as much as possible afterward. Heat can actually cause congestion, making matters worse.

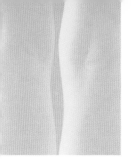

Osteoarthritis

Stiff, painful joints, which often become hard and swollen as the cartilage between the bones, which acts as a cushion, wears away; may affect any joint, but is common in the hips, knees, spine, and fingers.

steoarthritis is commonly seen as the result of long-term wear and tear on weight-bearing joints, often as the result of occupational or sporting activities. However, this is not the only cause; previous injury or fracture, damage to the cartilage (especially in the knee), previous infection, congenital deformity (such as spinal curvature), or bunions may also lead to osteoarthritis.

Prevention

Maintaining a sensible weight and avoiding activities likely to lead to stress-related arthritis are the key factors. Marathon running, relentless jogging, and high-impact aerobics can all damage joint surfaces.

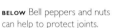

BELOW Bell peppers and nuts can help to protect joints.

 CONVENTIONAL MEDICINE

Try to stay as active as possible, which helps to keep the affected joints supple, increase muscle strength, and control weight gain, which can aggravate osteoarthritis. Staying active may mean taking pain relievers and using mechanical aids, such as a walking frame or stick. Your physician can arrange for physiotherapy, if required. In severe cases, a joint replacement can provide a new lease on life.

DOSAGE: ADULTS 1–2 tablets of pain relievers at onset of pain, repeated every 4 hours; consult label.

 NUTRITION

Oily fish are an important food group: the omega-3 fatty acids they contain are naturally anti-inflammatory and help to maintain joint mobility. Eat plenty of liver, carrots, spinach, broccoli, apricots, mangoes, and cantaloupe melons for their vitamin A and beta-carotene, which are equally important nutrients; all the green leafy vegetables, citrus fruits, kiwis, red, yellow and green bell peppers for their vitamin C, which helps to protect the joints from further damage. Avoid red meat and meat products as far as possible—instead, use fish, poultry, nuts, seeds, and beans, together with eggs and modest amounts of low-fat dairy products, as protein sources. Ginger tea can be soothing (avoid if you have gallstones). Peel and grate ½in/1cm of fresh ginger root, add to a mug of boiling water, cover for 10 minutes. Strain and add 1 tsp of honey (not for children under two).

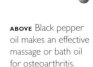

 HERBAL REMEDIES

A number of herbs may help this condition.

USE AND DOSAGE "Wear and tear" contributing to osteoarthritis may be eased by use of comfrey cream or oil (avoid if you are pregnant or breast-feeding): massage a little into the aching joint every night for at least 2 months.

Internally, herbs to stimulate circulation and clear toxins can help—try a decoction of angelica, yellow dock, and willow bark (1–2tsp per cup).

ABOVE Black pepper oil makes an effective massage or bath oil for osteoarthritis.

HOMEOPATHIC REMEDIES

A consultation with a homeopath is recommended.

Rhus toxicodendron 6c

For tearing pains, worse at night, restless with them. Pain worse for initial movement, then improves as gets moving. Joints feel sore and stiff. Worse for wet or cold weather.

Pulsatilla 6c

For pains that are wandering from joint to joint. Weepy with the pains and emotional. Pains better for gentle motion. Worse for warmth.

DOSAGE 1 tablet three times daily. Maximum 2 weeks.

AROMATHERAPY

Lavender (*Lavandula angustifolia*)
Roman chamomile (*Chamaemelum nobile*)
Marjoram (*Origanum majorana*)
Black pepper (*Piper nigrum*)
Rosemary (*Rosmarinus officinalis*)
Juniper (*Juniperus communis*)

Avoid rosemary and juniper if you are pregnant and juniper if you have a kidney problem. Do not give marjoram to babies or small children.

APPLICATION Use in warm baths and in hand or foot baths. Add to massage oils or lotions, but do not massage over any inflamed area.

Osteoporosis

Characterized by a weakening of the bones, loss of height, and a stooped posture; although it often does not produce symptoms, it is the most common cause of fractures in people over the age of 75; carries a strong familial link.

steoporosis—a condition in which bones become weak and brittle and break easily—normally occurs in women after menopause, though men can get it, too. It is increasing at an alarming rate and must be seen as an extremely serious problem. Any medical condition that causes a premature menopause (see p.110) increases the risk of osteoporosis; so does long-term treatment with certain drugs as well as eating disorders like anorexia and bulimia. Diseases that affect the body's absorption of nutrients—particularly Crohn's disease, colitis, and diverticulitis—also increase risk.

BELOW Weight-bearing exercise is fundamental to the prevention of osteoporosis.

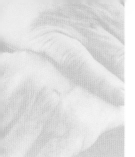

 CONVENTIONAL MEDICINE

To reduce the risk of osteoporosis, encourage children to perform regular weight-bearing exercise and to have a diet rich in calcium. Older women are advised to increase their calcium and vitamin D intake through diet and supplements. Avoid smoking and excessive consumption of alcohol and caffeine. Hormone replacement therapy helps prevent osteoporosis and can be taken at any stage after menopause, usually for at least 5 years. Existing osteoporosis can be treated with prescribed drugs. Keep exercising to maintain bone strength.

 HOMEOPATHIC REMEDIES

In homeopathy the patient is treated according to the symptoms that the body produces. Osteoporosis often does not produce symptoms until a fracture occurs, so there are no specific remedies.

 NUTRITION

The key to avoiding osteoporosis is building strong bones from the teens onward, but sadly this is also the time when many girls get on the dieting treadmill. A low calcium intake in the early years is almost a guarantee of bone problems later on. The average moderately active woman needs around 2,000 calories per day; it is impossible to get all the nutrients you need for strong bones on very low-calorie diets (under 1,250 calories per day).

The diet of all women should be rich in foods that contain calcium, vitamin D, bioflavonoids, vitamin K, and magnesium. For calcium, eat low-fat dairy products, nuts and sesame seeds, beans, and sardines (with their bones); for vitamin D, eat eggs and oily fish; for vitamin C and bioflavonoids eat citrus fruits, blackcurrants, blueberries, and blackberries; for vitamin K, eat spinach, broccoli, and cabbage; eat tofu, almonds, and cashews for their magnesium. Limit your intake of calcium-depleting foods such as sugar, salt, caffeine, alcohol, and meat.

BLACKBERRIES

ABOVE Vitamin D, found in oily fish, is needed for the absorption of calcium.

AROMATHERAPY

- Fennel *(Foeniculum vulgare)*
- Black pepper *(Piper nigrum)*
- Rosemary *(Rosmarinus officinalis)*
- Lavender *(Lavandula angustifolia)*
- Roman chamomile *(Chamaemelum nobile)*
- Marjoram *(Origanum majorana)*
- Benzoin *(Styrax benzoin)*

These oils are warming, soothing, and anti-inflammatory. Fennel contains plant estrogens.
APPLICATION Use in baths, foot baths, or bowls of warm water. They can also be massaged in.

HERBAL REMEDIES

Herbs rich in minerals, vitamins, and steroidal compounds are recommended to combat bone loss in old age and can contribute greatly to dietary needs.
USE AND DOSAGE Drink a daily tea of stinging nettles, alfalfa, and sage (2tsp per cup) and take 2tsp of horsetail juice in water three times daily. Dong Quai also provides nourishment. (Avoid sage and Dong Quai if pregnant and horsetail and stinging nettle if you have a heart or kidney problem.)

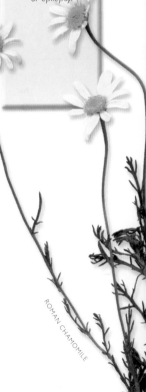

Caution
Do not use rosemary or fennel oil if you are pregnant, have high blood pressure, or epilepsy.

ROMAN CHAMOMILE

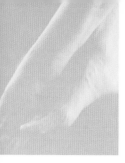

Rheumatism

Characterized by general aches and pains that affect the muscles, tendons, and connective tissue—often, but not always, surrounding the joints; may be accompanied by stiffness.

Rheumatism is a vague and general term describing aching joints or muscles, but it is not a specific disease. Repetitive strain injury (RSI) *(see p.76)*, tennis elbow, frozen shoulder, and tendonitis are just some of the disorders that can be grouped together under the broad heading of rheumatism. Even fibrositis is part of this collection. None of them is linked to osteoarthritis or rheumatoid arthritis. Your physician may offer you anti-inflammatory drugs or even steroid injections, but there are home remedies that may be just as effective. Unless you are in severe pain, try these first, as none of them has any side-effects.

 Call the physician

If your symptoms persist for a period of longer than 3–4 weeks.

Caution

Do not use rosemary oil if you are pregnant, or suffer from high blood pressure or epilepsy.

 CONVENTIONAL MEDICINE

Often resting for a few days, followed by gentle stretching exercises, is all that is required. A warm hot-water bottle, castor oil pack, or ice pack can help. Some people find that a firm supportive bandage provides enormous relief. Take pain relievers as required. Your physician may want to arrange for further investigations if the symptoms persist.

DOSAGE: ADULTS 1–2 tablets of pain relievers at onset of pain, repeated every 4 hours; consult label.

DOSAGE: CHILDREN Treat children only on the advice of a physician.

 AROMATHERAPY

- Lavender *(Lavandula angustifolia)*
- Roman chamomile *(Chamaemelum nobile)*
- Marjoram *(Origanum majorana)*
- Ginger *(Zingiber officinale)*
- Benzoin *(Styrax benzoin)*
- Rosemary *(Rosmarinus officinalis)*

Some of these oils may be more beneficial to you than others. Avoid rosemary if you are pregnant and do not use ginger if you have gallstones. Do not use marjoram for babies or small children.

APPLICATION Use in the bath (except benzoin), or in a compress. You can also use them in a massage: never massage over swollen and inflamed joints; massage over the affected area between flare-ups.

HERBAL REMEDIES

Anti-inflammatory rubs (such as 5 drops of chamomile essence in 1tsp of infused St. John's wort oil) can be helpful for tennis elbow or frozen shoulder when they are massaged over the affected area. Rheumatism may also respond to cleansing teas, which remove toxins that are located in the tissues.

USE AND DOSAGE Try an infusion of meadowsweet (do not use if you are sensitive to aspirin), and yarrow leaves (2tsp).

HOMEOPATHIC REMEDIES

If the following do not help, consult a homeopath.

Colchicum 6c

For severe inflammation of joints, with severe pain. Person is irritable. Worse for any motion. May affect several joints at once, or move from left to right side. Worse at night. Also used for gout.

Dulcamara 6c

For stiff and painful joints. Worse in autumn, for cold and damp, getting wet. Better for moving, dry weather. May also have diarrhea.

DOSAGE 1 tablet three times daily. Maximum 2 weeks.

NUTRITION

Eat plenty of oily fish and all the powerful antioxidant foods, which are rich in vitamins A, C, and E (see Arthritis on p.66) and in the minerals zinc and selenium. Use celery seeds (not celery salt) liberally in cooking. Avoid foods that will aggravate your inflammation, like red meat; and those likely to increase your levels of uric acid, such as organ meat, yeast, yeast extracts, meat extracts, roe, and even caviar; avoid all red and fortified wines, and drink other forms of alcohol in moderation. Do not drink more than 1–2 cups of coffee a day.

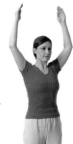
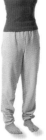

LEFT To benefit shoulders, elbows, and knees, stand tall and raise your hands above your head.

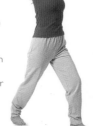

RIGHT Step forward with one foot, keeping your hands high. Hold, then repeat on the other side.

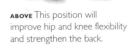

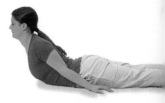

ABOVE This position will improve hip and knee flexibility and strengthen the back.

ABOVE Raising the chest while keeping the hips on the floor preserves mobility and strength in the spine.

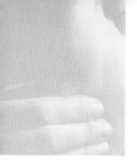

Cramp

Sudden and continuous pain in a muscle, often the calf or foot, although it can flare up anywhere in the body; the pain, caused by involuntary contraction of the muscle, may develop during exercise or at night.

This sudden condition always seems to strike at the most inappropriate moments. It is most common in the calf muscles and is excruciatingly uncomfortable, often leaving you feeling as though you have been kicked by a mule. The common wisdom is that it is due to a deficiency of salt, but this is hardly ever the case. Potassium deficiency is a far more likely cause. Cramp can also occur if the muscles are not receiving enough oxygen because the blood supply is impaired. Cramps at night are common in pregnant women and the elderly, although they may be a sign of a more serious underlying condition, such as diabetes.

 Call the physician
If you have experienced pain in the chest or calves during exercise.

Prevention
Occupational cramps are caused by relentless but controlled repetitive movements. Practice some relaxation techniques and take regular breaks.

 CONVENTIONAL MEDICINE

Cramp-like pain will usually go away when the muscle is relaxed. This generally means resting for a few minutes. Cramps at night are often relieved by stretching and rubbing the affected muscle. Pain in the chest or calves during exercise, which stops after resting, can be more serious and may require medical attention.

 NUTRITION

Nutrition is often the key to relieving attacks of cramp, but it must be seen as a long-term benefit, and not as an instant cure. If you suffer regularly from cramp, eat at least one banana each day for the potassium that it contains. Vitamin E is a great aid to the circulation, so eat avocados, nuts, seeds and lots of good olive oil. Sardines contain beneficial omega-3 fatty acids and also are a rich source of calcium, as are all dairy products. Eat natural yogurt for its riboflavin and eggs for their vitamin B_{12}. A glass of tonic water taken at bedtime—without the gin—often helps, due to its quinine content.

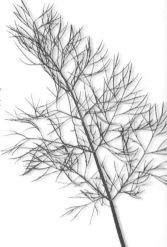

To help alleviate or prevent cramp take 400 IU of vitamin E each day and a good mineral supplement containing calcium, potassium, and magnesium.

 HOMEOPATHIC REMEDIES

❧ **Cuprum metallicum 6c**
For violent, sudden cramps in the calves at night. Useful for cramps that occur during pregnancy. Try this remedy first.

❧ **Magnesium phosphoricum 6c**
For writer's cramp, cramps from prolonged exertion. Cramps in the calves better for rubbing.

❧ **Nux vomica 6c**
For cramps in the calves and soles, with lots of muscle spasms. Sleeplessness, particularly toward morning, with dreams of arguments. Person may be irritable.

DOSAGE 1 tablet before retiring. Maximum 2 weeks.

 HERBAL REMEDIES

Decoctions (see p.187) of cramp bark or black haw can help night cramp. Teas of wild yam, chamomile, or fennel (avoid if pregnant) ease stomach cramps.

USE AND DOSAGE Add 1tsp of cramp bark or black haw to 1½ cups/350ml of water, simmer for 10 minutes. Make an external rub using 5 drops each of cypress, marjoram, and basil oils in 1tbsp of almond oil. (Avoid cypress and basil if pregnant. Do not use marjoram for babies or small children.)

AROMATHERAPY

❧ **Geranium** (Pelargonium graveolens)
❧ **Ginger** (Zingiber officinale)
❧ **Cypress** (Cupressus sempervirens)
These oils are stimulating and increase circulation, warming up the muscles so that cramp does not set in. (Avoid cypress if pregnant; ginger if you have gallstones.)

APPLICATION Use in a compress, in the bath, or in a foot spa. You should be looking at prevention, rather than cure, so massage the feet and legs in the evenings, before you go to bed.

BELOW Cypress oil helps to ease the pain caused by cramp.

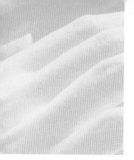

Repetitive strain injury: RSI

Pain in the hand, wrist, forearm, shoulder, and/or neck, often related to using a keyboard for long periods, although any repetitive task may bring it on.

MEADOWSWEET

epetitive strain injury is a result of overuse of the upper body at work, and should properly be called work-related upper-limb injury. The best treatment may be rest and home remedies.

CONVENTIONAL MEDICINE

Make sure your keyboard, monitor, and desk are comfortable and ergonomically safe. Take regular breaks, and rest until any pain has gone completely. If it persists, try a non-steroidal anti-inflammatory pain reliever, such as aspirin or ibuprofen. Your physician may suggest that you see a specialist.

DOSAGE: ADULTS 1–2 tablets of pain relievers at onset of pain, repeated every 4 hours; consult label.

HERBAL REMEDIES

Anti-inflammatory herbs like meadowsweet (do not use if you are sensitive to aspirin) or St. John's wort may be helpful in teas.

USE AND DOSAGE Use 2tsp of these herbs per cup.

Herbal rubs for rheumatism *(see p.72)* and arthritis *(see p.66)* may provide relief.

Siberian ginseng may improve chronic cases.

HOMEOPATHIC REMEDIES

Arnica 6c

For bruised sensation in muscles and tendons. Aching muscles after overexertion. Worse for damp weather and continuing movement. Person says he or she is fine, even when obviously not.

Causticum 6c

For burning pain, inflamed tendons. Pain worse for drafts, cold, or overuse. Carpal tunnel syndrome. Person is very idealistic and intense.

DOSAGE 1 tablet twice daily. Maximum 2 weeks.

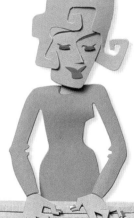

ABOVE Typists not trained to work with the correct posture might find a wrist support helpful.

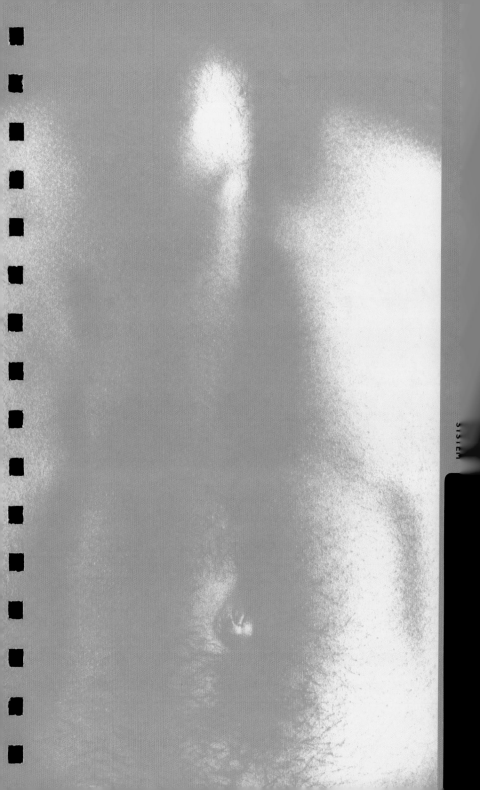

The Digestive System

Digestion enables the body to convert the food that we eat into energy and use it to build and repair tissues. A healthy digestive system is vital for general well-being, but in our rushed modern lifestyles it is often abused, leading to many of the problems that plague our daily lives, from indigestion and abdominal pain to peptic ulcers and gastroenteritis. Weight concerns—either too much or too little—are another manifestation of digestive problems. But with a little thought and a sensible diet, many of these ailments can be treated.

Heartburn

Burning sensation in upper abdomen, going up the center of the chest to the back of the throat, often with an acid taste in the mouth; pain may be worse at night, when lying flat, bending, or stooping.

Heartburn, also known as acid indigestion, may be caused by obesity, the late stages of pregnancy or a hiatus hernia, but most often results from too much of the wrong kind of food or plain overeating. The acid contents of the stomach escape upward into the esophagus, causing the characteristic burning sensation behind the breastbone. Whatever the cause, home remedies can help resolve the discomfort.

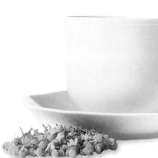

ABOVE Herbal teas containing caraway, cardamom, ginger, or tangerine can help relieve heartburn.

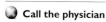
Call the physician

If heartburn continues for a long period of time, as it can be indicative of complaints such as ulcers or gallstones; if the symptoms persist or are not relieved by an antacid.

CONVENTIONAL MEDICINE

Avoid eating fatty foods or consuming hot drinks or alcohol. Try to stop smoking, and lose weight if necessary. If the symptoms are worse at night, try raising the head of the bed by 2–3in/5–7cm. Take an antacid if the symptoms continue.

DOSAGE: ADULTS AND CHILDREN OVER 16 Many types of antacid are available in tablet or liquid form. Be aware that they contain magnesium or aluminum salts, or both: the former (e.g. Milk of Magnesia) tend to cause diarrhea; the latter (e.g. Aluminum hydroxide) constipation. Some antacids are combined with alginic acid and are particularly helpful for heartburn; consult label for details.

HERBAL REMEDIES

Soothing herbs, such as marshmallow, ginger (avoid if you have gallstones), and slippery elm, are widely used for heartburn.

USE AND DOSAGE Take these herbs in tablets or capsules (200mg) before meals.

Teas of antacid herbs, such as centaury (avoid if you have an ulcer) or black horehound, can be useful. Carminative (anti-gas) teas for indigestion *(see p.80)* may help, or make a thin gruel by mixing 1tsp of powdered slippery-elm bark with a little water, then add a hot chamomile infusion.

HOMEOPATHIC REMEDIES

Persistent heartburn requires medical assessment, but a consultation with a homeopath may help.

🐾 Robina 6c

For heartburn with acidity. Worse at night and for lying down. Prevents sleep. Abdomen bloated with wind and colic. Headaches.

🐾 Sulphur 6c

For heartburn from eating either too much, or spicy, food. Big appetite, craves spices, alcohol, fats. Thirsty for cold drinks.

DOSAGE 1 tablet hourly for six doses. May be repeated if necessary.

🍎 NUTRITION

Avoiding the symptoms of heartburn is simply a matter of applying common sense to your eating habits. Avoid alcohol, nicotine, and caffeine. Do not overeat or eat very acidic or irritant foods, such as chilis (avoid if pregnant), pickles, raw onion, sour fruit, very hot curries, or deep-fried foods. If you have a hiatus hernia or are in the later stages of pregnancy, make sure that you eat little and often, spreading your daily intake over five meals instead of three. Use all the good digestive herbs routinely—mint, dill, ginger (avoid if you have gallstones), and slippery elm *(see Gastritis on p.104)*—and end your meals with a glass of mint tea. Heartburn sometimes responds well to a few weeks on the food combining (Hay) diet *(see p.200)*.

🌼 AROMATHERAPY

🐾 Fennel *(Foeniculum vulgare)*
🐾 Peppermint *(Mentha piperita)*
🐾 Black pepper *(Piper nigrum)*
🐾 Roman chamomile *(Chamaemelum nobile)*

These oils calm and soothe the digestive tract. (Avoid fennel if pregnant and peppermint if you have a gallbladder or liver problem.)

APPLICATION Use in a massage oil or lotion.

Prevention

Obesity is a major—and in many cases, a controllable—cause of heartburn. Simply losing weight and avoiding tight, restrictive clothes will make an enormous difference.

Caution

If you are pregnant, do not take any medicines without first consulting your physician.

BELOW Sometimes heartburn can be eased by following the principles of food combining.

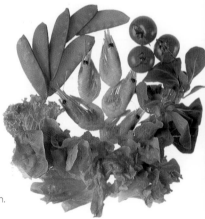

Indigestion

Pain or discomfort experienced in the upper part of the abdomen, related to food; it may be associated with nausea and belching; the tendency to indigestion often increases with age.

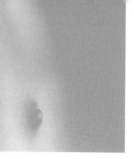

There cannot be a single person who has not had the occasional bout of indigestion, and except when underlying diseases are involved, indigestion is always self-inflicted. Indigestion starts in the kitchen and that is where you will find the solution.

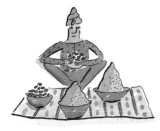

CONVENTIONAL MEDICINE

Don't eat right before bedtime, and avoid alcohol, cigarettes, and tight-fitting clothes. Raising the head of the bed may help.

When the pain starts, try drinking milk; if that does not help, take an antacid. If the symptoms of indigestion still do not respond to such measures, then a short course of cimetidine or ranitidine may help.

DOSAGE: ADULTS AND CHILDREN OVER 16 For information on antacids, *see Heartburn on p.78.* Other indigestion mixtures contain dimethicone to relieve gas; consult label for details.

Take an over-the-counter drug when heartburn symptoms appear or at least 30 minutes before you anticipate them. Read the labels for maximum daily dosages.

If symptoms persist or worsen, consult your physician. Avoid taking either cimetidine or ranitidine if you are pregnant.

 Call the physician

If you have a persistent problem with indigestion; if you have the symptoms and have lost weight unintentionally; if it is the first time you have had these symptoms and you are over 40 years old.

HERBAL REMEDIES

Carminative (anti-gas) herbs like caraway, cardamom, and ginger (avoid if you have gallstones) may help.

USE AND DOSAGE Make a standard infusion or use these herbs in tinctures (½tsp diluted with water, or up to 20 drops on the tongue).

Slippery elm or marshmallow-root capsules will help protect the stomach lining.

❖ HOMEOPATHIC REMEDIES

Persistent symptoms require medical attention, but a consultation with a homeopath may be helpful.

☙ Lycopodium 30c

For burning in throat. Pressure in stomach and bitter taste in mouth. Bloating immediately after meals. Craves warm drinks.

☙ Nux vomica 30c

For pain, like a stone, in the stomach some time after meals, together with nausea. Indigestion from drinking strong coffee.

☙ Carbo vegetabilis 30c

For heaviness, fullness, sleepiness after food. Food turns to gas in stomach, with belching and flatus.

DOSAGE 1 tablet hourly for six doses, then three times daily. Maximum 1 week.

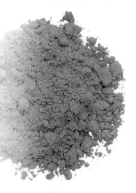

ABOVE Ginger is an established treatment for nausea and indigestion.

◐ AROMATHERAPY

☙ **Peppermint** *(Mentha x piperita)*
☙ **Black pepper** *(Piper nigrum)*
☙ **Roman chamomile** *(Chamaemelum nobile)*
☙ **Ginger** *(Zingiber officinale)*

These oils calm and soothe the digestive tract. Avoid ginger if you are pregnant and peppermint if you have a gallbladder or liver problem.

APPLICATION Use in a massage oil or lotion.

◍ NUTRITION

RADISHES

Long gaps between meals, eating on the run, large, rich meals late at night, and a surfeit of greasy or deep-fried food represent an assault on your digestive system. So eat a well-balanced diet with regular meals.

Avoid eating too much of the obvious culprits—raw onions, pickles, hot, spicy chili and curry, radishes, cucumber, and bell peppers; unripe bananas are particularly indigestible. A glass of mint tea is an almost instant cure—sweetened with a bit of honey (not for children under two), one of the great digestive soothers. Another traditional remedy is a generous pinch of baking soda dissolved on the tongue.

> **Caution**
> Severe pain after eating or when hungry, blood in the stool, and long-standing chronic digestive problems could be symptoms of a more serious condition. Avoid aspirin and NSAIDS, which may make the symptoms worse.

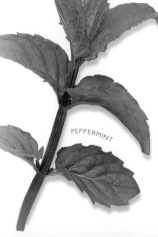
PEPPERMINT

Nausea

Sensation of impending vomiting, often accompanied by sweating, excessive salivation, dizziness, and pale skin; in pregnancy it tends to be worst in the first 3–4 months, but may continue throughout in rare cases, at any time of day.

ausea, that familiar feeling of sickness, may be followed by vomiting. This violent expulsion of the stomach contents may bring relief if the vomiting has been triggered by overindulgence or the ingestion of some toxic substance. But it may also be the first of a series of repeated bouts in a prolonged episode, if the underlying cause is food poisoning or some other form of infection *(see Gastroenteritis on p.102)*. High temperatures in children, appendicitis, motion sickness, pregnancy, migraine, liver and gallbladder disease, whooping cough, vertigo, Ménière's disease, and severe anxiety can all cause nausea.

BELOW So-called morning sickness can happen at any time of day, but can be relieved by small amounts of food, such as a ginger cookie.

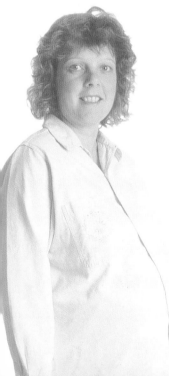

CONVENTIONAL MEDICINE

Avoid eating, but take frequent sips of plain water and lie down until the sensation passes. Antinausea treatments can be helpful, particularly for travel sickness, but consult your physician, as the remedy may depend on the cause of the nausea. Nausea due to pregnancy may be relieved by eating: try eating frequent light snacks throughout the day, possibly even before getting up in the morning.

DOSAGE: ADULTS AND CHILDREN   Treatments for travel sickness are usually taken before traveling and then repeated at regular intervals; consult label for details *(see also Motion Sickness on p.184)*.

HERBAL REMEDIES

Ginger is probably the most widely used herb for nausea *(see p.184)* (avoid if you have gallstones), but other useful remedies include chamomile, lemon balm, and bitter orange.

USE AND DOSAGE   Take these herbs in teas or, more easily during bouts of nausea, as drops of tincture (diluted 50:50 with water) on the tongue.

Black horehound can be very effective, but its distinctive flavor makes some people feel worse.

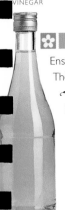

VINEGAR

✿ HOMEOPATHIC REMEDIES

Ensure there is no serious medical condition. These remedies are useful for morning sickness.

➣ Ipecacuanha 6c

For constant nausea, not relieved by vomiting. Clean tongue, needs to keep swallowing an excess of saliva.

➣ Sepia 6c

For nausea at sight, smell, or thought of food. Morning sickness before eating, vomits on rinsing mouth. Craves vinegar.

➣ Glossypium 6c

For nausea and vomiting worse before breakfast, movement, or standing up. No appetite, sensitive stomach with a lot of gas.

DOSAGE I tablet every half-hour. Maximum 12 doses.

> ### Caution
>
> *If you are pregnant, do not take any medicines without first consulting your physician. If you have glaucoma, do not take medicines containing hyoscine.*

💧 AROMATHERAPY

➣ Ginger (*Zingiber officinale*)
➣ Peppermint (*Mentha x piperita*)
➣ Lavender (*Lavandula angustifolia*)
➣ Roman chamomile (*Chamaemelum nobile*)

Peppermint acts as a mild anesthetic to the stomach wall (avoid if you have a gallbladder or liver problem); ginger is the universal remedy for nausea (avoid if you have gallstones.)

APPLICATION Use as a compress.

> ### 🌐 Call the physician
>
> *If nausea is a recurring problem; if bouts of nausea and vomiting have no obvious explanation; if you have been feeling nauseous for more than a week and you are not pregnant.*

🍽 NUTRITION

This depends on the cause of the nausea, but in general terms a bout of food poisoning should be treated with the BRAT diet (*see p.99*), followed by a gradual return to normal eating (*see Gastroenteritis on p.102*). Vomiting caused by ulcers needs a specific pattern of eating (*see Gastritis on p.104*). For nausea caused by vertigo or Ménière's disease follow the advice for motion sickness (*see p.184*). The young and elderly can dehydrate rapidly as a result of repeated vomiting—especially if accompanied by diarrhea. It is essential to replace lost fluids (*see p.102*).

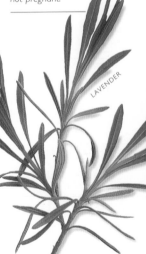

LAVENDER

Abdominal pain

*Waves of cramping pain, often with diarrhea and/or nausea—
likely cause: gastroenteritis; severe, constant pain in lower right
abdomen—likely cause: appendicitis; lower abdominal pain,
with pain on passing urine—likely cause: cystitis.*

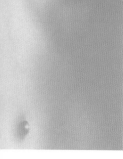

Abdominal pain (stomachache) is the result of abusing your
digestive system. Overindulgence, excessive alcohol, too much
fat, or unwise combinations of food may all be the culprit. It is a problem that most people will have occasionally; it can also be triggered by
stress and anxiety. Regular attacks of stomach pain need investigation
to rule out underlying disease. *(See also Constipation on p.96, Diarrhea
on p.98, Flatulence on p.86, Gallbladder Problems on p.88, Gastroenteritis
on p.102, Irritable Bowel Syndrome on p.94, Peptic Ulcers on p.92).*

BELOW Many causes of
abdominal pain can
be attributed to some
element of the diet.

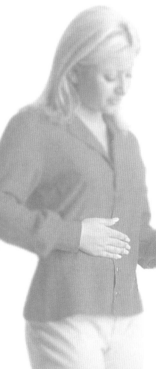

 CONVENTIONAL MEDICINE

Stomachache can initially be treated with a simple
pain reliever, such as acetaminophen (but not aspirin
or ibuprofen). Drink plenty of water, and eat only if
you are hungry. Avoid spicy or fatty foods until the
pain subsides. If it becomes worse, or remains
unchanged for several days, seek medical advice.
DOSAGE: ADULTS 1–2 tablets of pain relievers at
onset of pain, repeated every 4 hours; consult label
for details.
DOSAGE: CHILDREN Give regular doses of children's
pain relievers; consult label, or follow medical advice.

 HERBAL REMEDIES

Carminative (anti-gas) herbs—clove, coriander, fennel, parsley, and thyme—can help relieve the pain of
wind (avoid fennel and parsley if pregnant and
parsley if you have a heart or kidney condition).
Meadowsweet (do not use if you are sensitive to
aspirin) can ease inflammation associated with
overindulgence.
USE AND DOSAGE Use the herbs in standard infusions and decoctions; drink a cup every 3–4 hours.
Avoid laxative herbs if the cause of abdominal pain
is at all uncertain.

✿ HOMEOPATHIC REMEDIES

These remedies may also be used for infantile colic.

Magnesium phosphoricum 6c

For cramping abdominal pains. Better for heat, pulling legs up to abdomen, pressure, and rubbing. Belching gives no relief.

Dioscorea 6c

For colic pains. Better for stretching or for bending backward.

Colocynthis 6c

For cutting colic pains. Better for pressure, heat. Pains after anger. Bends over double; presses on abdomen for relief.

Chamomilla 6c

For infant colic. Greenish stool, infant's cry is angry, pains are unbearable. Better for being carried.

DOSAGE 1 tablet every half-hour. Maximum six doses.

◊ AROMATHERAPY

Lavender (*Lavandula angustifolia*)

Roman chamomile (*Chamaemelum nobile*)

Both oils are soothing and help to kill the pain.

APPLICATION Place a warm compress on the stomach and possibly on the lower back. A hot-water bottle can be used on top of the compress. If the pain continues and the reason is unknown, then good diagnosis is important. If the pain is due to constipation, gentle circular massage of the abdomen with lavender and chamomile will help.

🍎 NUTRITION

Everyone knows the proverb "You are what you eat," and this is true in relation to all digestive problems. Eat plenty of foods containing soluble fiber, such as oats, apples, pears, root vegetables, and all the bean family. When cooking vegetables, add a few caraway seeds; chew a few dill seeds and drink mint tea after meals. Reduce your intake of alcohol, coffee, and all carbonated drinks. Eat little and often and, cut down on all animal fats. A few weeks on the food combining (Hay) diet (*see p.200*) often works wonders for chronic digestive difficulties.

Caution

Avoid taking aspirin or ibuprofen, as they may irritate an already sore stomach lining. If using essential oils on small children, make sure that the doses are the relevant sizes.

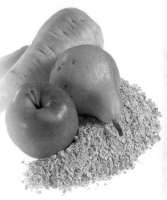

ABOVE Plenty of soluble fiber is essential to the efficient working of the digestive system.

 Call the physician

If pain becomes more severe, is associated with a fever, or has lasted more than a day or two; if you are in severe pain and unable to hold down fluids for more than 12 hours; if a child has severe abdominal pain.

Flatulence

Excessive gas, either through the mouth or through the anus, as a byproduct of the digestive process; often associated with a bloated feeling in the abdomen.

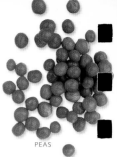
PEAS

omedians joke about it, yet nothing could be more natural than flatulence—the normal byproduct of digestion and fermentation that takes place in the gut. Many people feel obsessive anxiety about flatulence, but unless it becomes excessive there is no need for concern. Any sudden change in the everyday buildup and release of these gases could, however, herald an underlying problem. Possible causes are hiatus hernia, Irritable Bowel Syndrome *(see p.94)*, diverticulitis, or severe constipation *(see p.96)*. But in the absence of other disease, home remedies will usually overcome this problem.

BELOW Small changes in diet can bring about relief from excessive flatulence.

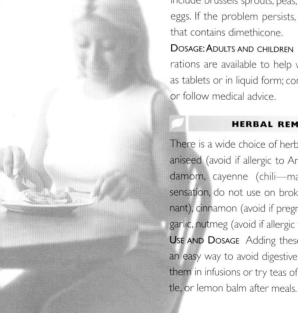

✚ CONVENTIONAL MEDICINE

A change in diet can be helpful, especially cutting down on beans, lentils, and other legumes. Other foods that could be reduced include brussels sprouts, peas, cabbage, and eggs. If the problem persists, try taking an antacid that contains dimethicone.

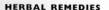
SPROUTS

DOSAGE: ADULTS AND CHILDREN Many suitable preparations are available to help with flatulence, either as tablets or in liquid form; consult labels for details, or follow medical advice.

🌿 HERBAL REMEDIES

There is a wide choice of herbal remedies including: aniseed (avoid if allergic to Anise or anethole), cardamom, cayenne (chili—may cause a burning sensation, do not use on broken skin; avoid if pregnant), cinnamon (avoid if pregnant), clove, coriander, garlic, nutmeg (avoid if allergic to nuts), and thyme. USE AND DOSAGE Adding these herbs to cooking is an easy way to avoid digestive problems. Also, drink them in infusions or try teas of chamomile, holy thistle, or lemon balm after meals.

HOMEOPATHIC REMEDIES

🜋 **Lycopodium 6c**

For bloating, better for passing wind. Rumbling in stomach. Eating little gives sense of fullness.

🜋 **Carbo vegetabilis 6c**

For heaviness after meals, sleepiness, and belching. Flatus smells offensive. Craves sweet and salt foods.

DOSAGE 1 tablet hourly for six doses, then twice daily. Maximum 1 week.

 AROMATHERAPY

🜋 **Roman chamomile** *(Chamaemelum nobile)*
🜋 **Fennel** *(Foeniculum vulgare)*
🜋 **Ginger** *(Zingiber officinale)*
🜋 **Peppermint** *(Mentha x piperita)*

These oils aid gas dispersal. Avoid fennel if you are pregnant; ginger if you have gallstones; peppermint if you have a gallbladder or liver problem.

APPLICATION Use in either an oil-based or lotion-based massage and rub onto the abdomen.

NUTRITION

To prevent flatulence, you must allow time for the digestive process to work—sit down to eat, savor your food, and chew it well. Avoid carbonated drinks, and don't drink while eating. Reduce your intake of sugar in all forms; also avoid beans, brussels sprouts, cauliflower, and other "windy" foods. As your eating habits improve and you add to your diet more live yogurt and other fermented milk products, with all their beneficial bacteria, you will find that you can return to eating virtually anything. It helps, too, if you add caraway seeds when cooking cabbage, and summer savory to all bean dishes. Dill, fennel seeds, licorice, and mint can be added to cooking and taken as tea, to prevent and relieve excessive gas. (Avoid fennel and licorice if pregnant and licorice if you have a liver or kidney problem.)

Constipation *(see p.96)* is an extremely common cause of gas and will be exacerbated if you start adding bran to your daily food intake. Instead, eat foods that contain soluble fiber, such as oats.

Prevention
Food combining, also known as the Hay diet (see p.200), which involves separating protein foods (like meat, fish, cheese, and eggs) from starchy foods (like bread, potatoes, rice, pasta, cereals, cookies, and cakes), may be a long-term solution for some people suffering from flatulence.

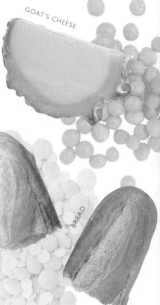

ABOVE Food combining may help: its principles state that bread and cheese should not be eaten together, but neutral foods like peas and lentils can be eaten with anything.

Gallbladder problems

Gallstones may not produce any symptoms, but can cause recurrent, painful attacks in the upper right abdomen; jaundice, with the whites of the eyes and skin appearing yellow; pain associated with fever; nausea is common.

The risk factors for the developments of gallstones are obesity, increasing age, and female gender (women are twice as likely as men to get them). At their worst, gallstones can block the flow of bile from the gallbladder to the stomach and, without bile, the digestion of fats becomes almost impossible. Then the sometimes horrendous symptoms of projectile vomiting and violent pain may ensue. However, home remedies can prevent problems recurring.

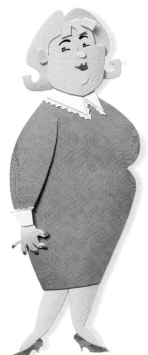

ABOVE Women are much more likely than men to be susceptible to gallstones.

CONVENTIONAL MEDICINE

If the pain from a gallstone continues, despite taking pain relievers, contact a physician. Seek immediate medical help if it is associated with fever or jaundice.
DOSAGE: ADULTS 1–2 tablets of pain relievers at onset of pain, repeated every 4 hours; consult label.

HERBAL REMEDIES

Professional help is essential for severe or persistent problems, but general discomfort can be soothed by anti-inflammatory and bitter herbs.
USE AND DOSAGE A traditional remedy for gallstones is a "liver-gall bladder flush." After breakfast, fast until early evening, then drink 2–4tbsp of olive oil, followed by the juice of 1–2 lemons diluted with as little warm water as possible. Alternate olive oil and lemon juice every 20–30 minutes until you have consumed 2 cups of olive oil and the juice of about 9–10 lemons. The gallstones should pass with stools over the next 3 days. Do not try a flush if you have gallbladder inflammation (cholecystitis).

Try decoctions of milk-thistle seeds or wild-yam root (1tsp per cup), or an infusion of fumitory and agrimony (1tsp each per cup).

Bitters before meals (2–5 drops of gentian or wormwood tincture) encourage bile flow.

HOMEOPATHIC REMEDIES

Consult a physician for gallbladder problems.

 Chelidonium 6c

For pain under right ribs extending to right shoulder blade. Colic, jaundice, gallstones, "bilious vomiting." Stools pasty/yellow.

Berberis 6c

For pain under right ribs radiating to stomach and all over body. Worse for pressure. Watery stools that are clay-colored.

Hydrastis 6c

For gallstones, tenderness over liver. No appetite or thirst. Jaundice. Stools white.

DOSAGE I tablet every 2–3 hours for six doses, then three times daily for 2–3 days.

AROMATHERAPY

Lavender *(Lavandula angustifolia)*

Roman chamomile *(Chamaemelum nobile)*

These oils help to reduce the pain.

APPLICATION Use in a massage oil or lotion, then apply over the area of the gallbladder.

NUTRITION

A problem gallbladder requires a strict diet, high in fiber and low in fat. To help dilute built-up gallbladder fluids, make sure to eat breakfast every day. Eat plenty of vegetables, fruit, and whole grain cereals; fish (avoid smoked fish); and beans. Have at least one large garlic clove (or a high-strength garlic pill) daily. Try to eat fresh globe artichokes at least two or three times a week—its chemicals have a specific stimulating effect on the gallbladder and liver.

Avoid alcohol and caffeine, but drink a minimum of 8 glasses of water, in addition to other drinks, daily. Avoid animal fats (no beef, pork, lamb, duck, or goose). Roasted (unbasted), grilled, or boiled chicken without skin is all right. Eat no butter, cream, cheese (except cottage cheese), eggs, or fried food. You can use skim milk, low-fat yogurt, and a little olive, sunflower or safflower oil. Do not eat pâté, sausages, salami, ham, bacon, or processed meat.

 Call the physician

If pain persists, especially if there is jaundice, a raised temperature, or protracted vomiting.

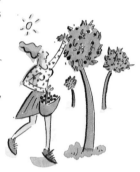

Caution

Always read pain reliever labels carefully, and do not exceed the stated dose.

BELOW Salmon can be a part of the strict diet necessary with gallbladder problems.

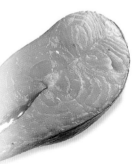

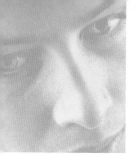

Worms and parasites

Parasitic skin infections may be characterized by small, red itchy blisters and severe itching, often worse at night; worms in the digestive tract may be passed in the stool and cause itching around the anus.

Parasites, such as head lice and scabies, and the wide variety of intestinal worms, such as pinworm, are no respecters of person or position. Intestinal parasites require medical attention, while skin infestations can take several treatments to clear, particularly in the case of head lice, which have become resistant to some currently available medicated shampoos and treatment lotions.

 Call the physician

If you suspect that you are suffering from an intestinal parasite.

Prevention

Most worms survive only in raw or undercooked food, so try to eat properly cooked food when abroad. The only way to protect yourself against head lice is never to let your hair come into direct contact with anyone else's.

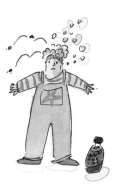

✚ CONVENTIONAL MEDICINE

Pinworms are easily treated with a single dose of mebendazole, available at your pharmacy, but make sure you treat the whole family. Parasitic skin infestations can be treated with insecticides, available as lotions and shampoos (treat the whole area). Do not use insecticides too often on children; instead, for head lice, regularly comb the hair with a fine nit-comb after washing. Apply conditioner and leave for 5 minutes before combing, then wash off.

DOSAGE: ADULTS AND CHILDREN For scabies, apply a water-based solution all over the body.

For head lice, apply a water-based lotion to the whole scalp. Repeat after 7 days.

For pinworms, take one dose of mebendazole, repeated 2 weeks later.

HERBAL REMEDIES

Cabbage is a traditional remedy for pinworms and can be used like carrots *(see under Nutrition)*. Take garlic as a preventative when traveling.

USE AND DOSAGE Wormwood is effective, but is very bitter: 1tsp (¼tsp for children) of the tincture, well diluted in water or carrot juice and taken on an empty stomach, may be sufficient to clear the problem. Repeat after 14 days (to match the pinworm's life cycle).

❖ HOMEOPATHIC REMEDIES

The following remedies should help to clear worms. If the symptoms persist, consult a physician.

◈ Cina 6c
Common name: wormseed. For patient who is restless and irritable. Itchy rectum. May have diarrhea and cramping abdominal pain, better for pressure.

◈ Sabadilla 6c
For chilly and not thirsty person. Itching in the rectum may alternate with itchy nose.

DOSAGE 1 tablet twice daily. Maximum 1 week.

◈ Staphysagria
For head lice, dilute mother tincture (available at homeopathic pharmacies) in a ratio of 1:10 with baby shampoo. Shampoo the hair, then leave on for 10 minutes, rinse and comb hair through. Repeat next night if there are further signs of lice. Repeat again 1 week later.

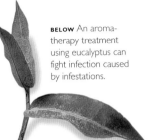

BELOW An aroma-therapy treatment using eucalyptus can fight infection caused by infestations.

◐ AROMATHERAPY

- ◈ Rosemary *(Rosmarinus officinalis)*
- ◈ Lavender *(Lavandula angustifolia)*
- ◈ Roman chamomile *(Chamaemelum nobile)*
- ◈ Niaouli *(Melaleuca viridiflora)*
- ◈ Eucalyptus *(Eucalyptus radiata)*
- ◈ Tea tree *(Melaleuca alternifolia)*

These oils are soothing and help to fight infection. Avoid rosemary if pregnant or breastfeeding. Avoid eucalyptus if you have digestive problems or liver disease; do not give to infants or small children.

APPLICATION For pinworm, massage the oils into the abdomen. This should be accompanied by treatment from your physician. For head lice, add 1–2 drops of the oils to the final rinse; or mix 2–3 drops with 1 tsp warm vegetable oil, massage into the hair, wrap in a plastic wrap and a warm towel, and leave overnight.

Caution
Asthmatics should avoid using alcoholic solutions for head lice; do not use them on infants either.

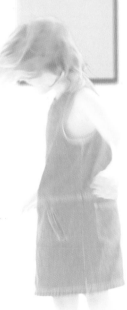

◉ NUTRITION

Eat a big portion of carrots or drink a large glass of carrot juice each day, to treat worms. Additionally, drink the juice of a whole lemon vigorously mixed with 1 tbsp of olive oil.

Peptic ulcers

Characterized by pain in the upper abdomen, often in a specific place, which may be pointed out with one finger; pain is often worse at night; it may also be worse when hungry and associated with nausea, flatulence, and heartburn.

Peptic ulcers are caused by erosion of the lining of the stomach by excessive amounts of gastric acid. While stress frequently plays a part, we now know that the balance between the acid digestive juices and the protective mucus produced by the stomach lining is also upset. The latest research has shown that bacteria called *Helicobacter pylori* cause most ulcers. These bacteria are very widespread and are common in cats, which may pass them on to their human owners.

Call the physician

If you have specific pain in the upper abdomen and have lost weight unintentionally; if it is the first time you have had these symptoms and you are over 40 years old; if the pain persists, despite symptomatic measures.

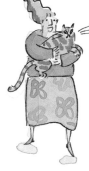

CONVENTIONAL MEDICINE

Avoid spicy foods, hot drinks, alcohol, and smoking. Do not take nonsteroidal anti-inflammatory drugs (NSAIDs), which are often used for pain relief. Eat frequent, regular, small meals of bland food. Antacids may help if symptoms persist for more than a week. Be aware they usually contain magnesium or aluminum salts: the former (e.g. Milk of Magnesia) tend to cause diarrhea; the latter (e.g. Aluminum hydroxide) constipation. Your physician may refer you for further tests. If you have *Helicobacter pylori* infection, you may need antibiotics.

DOSAGE: ADULTS AND CHILDREN OVER 16 Many types of antacid are available as tablets or in liquid form; consult labels for details.

HERBAL REMEDIES

Try herbal antibacterials, such as blue flag, wild iris, red clover, and thyme, in capsules or teas to combat the underlying cause. Symptomatic relief comes from soothing demulcents, such as slippery elm, marshmallow, or meadowsweet (do not take if you are sensitive to aspirin), taken in the form of teas, liquid extracts, or tinctures.

USE AND DOSAGE Mix 2tsp of slippery-elm powder with a cup of hot milk to make a gruel.

Dissolve licorice-juice sticks in water and take in 2tsp doses or add to teas. (Avoid licorice if pregnant or if you have a liver or kidney problem.)

 HOMEOPATHIC REMEDIES

A consultation with a homeopath is recommended, after seeing your physician.

Arsenicum album 6c

For raw, burning feeling in stomach. Worse for food and drink. Better for milk. Food feels as if it sticks in gullet, with nothing going through. Person is frightened and restless.

Phosphorus 6c

For burning pain. Worse for eating, better for cold food. Thirst for ice-cold water, but vomits soon afterward. May vomit "coffee grounds."

Dosage 1 tablet twice daily. Maximum 2 weeks.

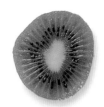

ABOVE A kiwi fruit contains twice as much vitamin C as an orange.

Caution

Non-steroidal anti-inflammatory drugs (NSAIDs) can make the symptoms worse.

 NUTRITION

Eat plenty of whole grains, pumpkin seeds, oysters, and most shellfish for their zinc; broccoli, red and green bell peppers, kiwis, apricots, and the sweeter citrus fruits for their vitamin C and beta-carotene; oily fish for its omega-3 fatty acids, which protect the whole gastric lining. A diet that is rich in fiber is also protective, but avoid spoonfuls of uncooked bran. Oats, brown rice, and most root vegetables contain soluble fiber, which is more soothing.

Scientists in New Zealand have shown that manuka honey (from the tea tree) can kill the bacteria responsible for ulcers: 2tsp with each meal and 2tsp at bedtime (but not for children under two) can produce results within a few weeks. In European natural medicine, raw cabbage juice and raw potato juice are known to be effective—take a small glass before each meal, on a daily alternating basis.

 AROMATHERAPY

The aim of aromatherapy here is to reduce stress levels, rather than treat the ulcer. So look up the oils for stress (see p.36). Make sure that you get a good diagnosis and that you really have a peptic ulcer.

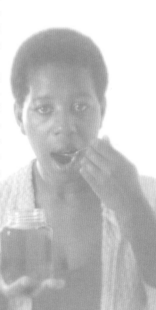

Irritable bowel syndrome: IBS

Recurrent episodes of abdominal pain with constipation or diarrhea; the pain is often relieved by passing wind or a bowel movement.

Irritable bowel syndrome has in recent years graduated from a relatively obscure condition, known as spastic colon, to one of near epidemic proportions throughout the US and Britain. Though it can be the sequel to a severe bout of food poisoning or gastroenteritis, it is far more likely to be the result of an overconsumption of bran fiber and underconsumption of the soluble fiber that is found in fruit and vegetables. It is not caused by the yeast infection *Candida*; nor is it, as many physicians believe, a symptom of depression or other psychological illness. Stress, however, can play a major part.

BELOW Antispasmodic drugs can alleviate the symptoms of IBS, but dietary changes will also be needed.

 CONVENTIONAL MEDICINE

Keeping a food diary can help to establish links between symptoms and particular foods. Relaxation techniques may be beneficial. If the symptoms persist, your physician may recommend medication to relax the muscle in the digestive tract.

 HERBAL REMEDIES

Herbs can help ease the discomfort of irritable bowel syndrome.

USE AND DOSAGE Make an infusion from equal amounts of agrimony, hops, meadowsweet (avoid if you are sensitive to aspirin), and peppermint (avoid if you have a gallbladder or liver problem) and drink a cup before meals.

Simmer 2tsp of fenugreek seeds with a pinch of cinnamon (avoid if pregnant) in water for 10–15 minutes, then drink.

 HOMEOPATHIC REMEDIES

If the following do not help, consult a homeopath.
Lycopodium 6c

For bloating, better for passing wind. Rumbling in stomach. Eating little gives a sense of fullness.

Craves candies, warm food and drink. Hard stool changes to liquid. Constipation away from home.

๑. Nux vomica 6c

For cramping abdominal pains. Worse for eating. Better after bowel movements and for warm drinks. Constipation: small amounts of stool. Constant feeling of need to go to toilet. Diarrhea alternates with constipation.

DOSAGE I tablet twice daily. Maximum I week.

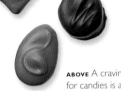

ABOVE A craving for candies is a symptom of some types of IBS.

AROMATHERAPY

๑. Neroli *(Citrus aurantium)*
๑. Roman chamomile *(Chamaemelum nobile)*
๑. Rose *(Rosa damascena/Rosa centifolia)*

These oils are calming and soothing.

APPLICATION Use in abdominal massage, with either an aqueous cream or oil. These oils can also be used in a warm compress or in the bath.

NUTRITION

If alternating bouts of constipation, diarrhea, flatulence, and stomach distension have been with you for years, do not despair. Changing your eating habits can restore your life to normal. Keep detailed records of what you eat and its effects, so that you know which foods are okay and which to avoid.

Eat plenty of food that contains soluble fiber—fruit, vegetables, beans, and especially oats. Cereals contain a mixture of soluble and insoluble fiber; wheat bran is not only an irritant, but can interfere with the way the body absorbs vital nutrients like iron and calcium. You must drink at least 6 cups of water every day and make sure that you eat proper meals at regular intervals. Use plenty of herbs that help digestion—sage (avoid if pregnant), thyme, mint, dill, caraway, and garlic.

For some people IBS is an adverse reaction to specific foods. These include: meat and meat products, milk and dairy foods, and corn or wheat products. Try excluding suspect foods in groups—one at a time, for at least 2 weeks to provide clues about which foods to avoid.

Prevention

Simple herbal remedies like hypericum have no side-effects, are not habit-forming, and will help with depression while you experiment with your diet.

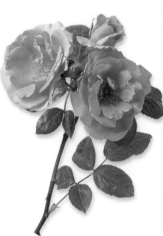

ABOVE Rose oil used in an abdominal massage can help to soothe pain and discomfort.

Constipation

PRUNES

Typified by a straining to defecate; hard feces that are sometimes painful to pass; stomach pain, bloating, and gas; and a general feeling of malaise.

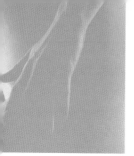

onstipation is one of the most common digestive problems, and the one that is most suited to home treatment. People vary as to how often they move their bowels: some maybe no more than every 2 or 3 days; others two or three times a day, or more often. Children, the elderly, and pregnant women are more prone to constipation, but it can occur in either sex at any age. A lack of the right sort of soluble fiber, insufficient fluid, and bad bathroom habits are the prime causes.

CONVENTIONAL MEDICINE

If the bowel has stretched and is full of feces, it needs retraining to respond to the urge to go to the bathroom regularly, without straining. Changing your diet and increasing your fluid intake may take a day or two to have any effect. In the meantime, a laxative and suppositories can help. If you suspect that prescribed medicines are causing your constipation, consult your physician before reducing the dose. If constipation persists seek medical help.

DOSAGE: ADULTS Natural or vegetable laxatives are safe and non-addictive, so ask your pharmacist for advice; consult labels for dosage information. One or two glycerol suppositories once a day, moistened before use, will stimulate bowel movement.

DOSAGE: CHILDREN See a physician about laxatives.

HERBAL REMEDIES

Do not use senna if you have an intestinal disorder and do not give to children under 12.

USE AND DOSAGE Each morning take a decoction of dandelion, yellow dock, and licorice roots (2tsp of each to 1½ cups of water). (Avoid licorice if pregnant or if you have a liver or kidney problem and dandelion if you have a bowel or gallbladder problem.)

Lubricate the bowel with a psyllium seed drink (avoid if you are diabetic)—add 1tsp to a cup of boiling water, allow to cool, then drink.

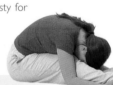

LEFT Sit tall with your legs straight out in front of you, then raise your arms above your head.

❀ HOMEOPATHIC REMEDIES

Sudden changes in bowel habit need medical attention.

∽ Alumina 6c

For soft, sticky or hard, dry stools that are difficult to pass, even when soft. Constipation in the elderly, from inactivity. No urge to move bowels.

∽ Bryonia 6c

For hard, dry, large crumbly stools. May have diarrhea after taking cold drinks. Thirsty for large quantities of fluids.

DOSAGE 1 tablet three times daily. Maximum 1 week.

BELOW Exhale and bend forward toward your feet, then lower your head and hold for several breaths.

🍎 NUTRITION

Drink at least 8 cups of water each day and eat unpeeled apples, pears, root vegetables, oats, beans, and all green vegetables; at least one carton of live natural yogurt daily; and plenty of real whole wheat bread, brown rice, whole wheat pasta, and muesli. Do not use uncooked bran or high-bran cereals.

LEFT Sit with your left arm around your right knee, with your right hand on the floor behind you.

For a gentle laxative pour 5 cups of boiling water over 2lb/1kg of stoned prunes and a few pieces of bruised licorice stick. Leave to stand overnight. Remove the licorice, then purée the prunes. Keep in the refrigerator and take 4tsp with breakfast and 4tsp with a warm drink at bedtime. (Avoid licorice if pregnant or if you have a liver or kidney problem.)

💧 AROMATHERAPY

∽ Black pepper *(Piper nigrum)*
∽ Marjoram *(Origanum majorana)*

These oils stimulate the digestive system.

APPLICATION Mix the essential oil with a lotion or a carrier oil and massage over the abdomen in a clockwise direction. Do not use marjoram for babies or small children.

LEFT Breathe out and turn to look behind you. Hold for several breaths, then repeat on the other side.

Diarrhea

Unusually frequent passing of feces which are often soft or watery, or may be more bulky than normal; there may also be symptoms reflecting the underlying cause of the diarrhea, including fever, vomiting, and cramp-like abdominal pain.

Diarrhea is a symptom, not an illness. The passing of frequent, loose, or even liquid stool (sometimes uncontrollable) is the result of irritation or inflammation of the gut. It is often accompanied by severe vomiting and may be caused by overindulgence, too much alcohol, or by bacterial infection from food poisoning. Most minor bouts can be dealt with adequately at home, but prolonged diarrhea may be the result of a more serious underlying illness and can cause severe dehydration, particularly in small children and the elderly.

🌐 Call the physician

If there is any sudden change in bowel habits that lasts more than 2–3 days (sooner in children and the elderly).

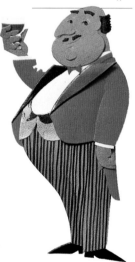

ABOVE Too much rich living can bring on an attack of diarrhea.

CONVENTIONAL MEDICINE

Water, salts, and minerals lost through diarrhea need to be replaced. This is particularly important in children and frail adults. Drinking extra water will help, but special oral rehydration fluid preparations are available. They can be flavored or made into ice cubes to make them more palatable. Prolonged diarrhea may require medical treatment, especially if there is blood, severe abdominal pain, or high fever. DOSAGE: ADULTS AND CHILDREN Dissolve the contents of an oral rehydration packet in water and drink after each episode of diarrhea. Consult label.

HERBAL REMEDIES

To soothe an inflamed digestive tract, drink unsweetened black tea: the high tannin content soothes and repairs sore tissues. Other herbs to use in teas include agrimony, bistort, lady's mantle, raspberry leaves, and tormentil (shepherd's knot). USE AND DOSAGE Use 2tsp of herb per cup of boiling water.

Pack a small bottle of tincture of any of these herbs to combat holiday diarrhea (take 1tsp in water up to six times a day), or eat some papaya—a traditional tropical remedy (avoid if pregnant).

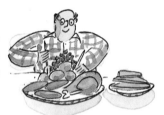

HOMEOPATHIC REMEDIES

Diarrhea requires the same general measures as for gastroenteritis *(see p.102).* Persistent diarrhea needs medical investigation. Many remedies are indicated, but these are among the most common.

⟶ Podophyllum 6c
Gushing, watery diarrhea. Stool may be pasty or yellow. Colic pains better for lying on abdomen.

⟶ China 6c
For painless diarrhea of undigested food, flatulence, and colic. Worse after eating fruit. Patient feels weak.

⟶ **Dosage** I tablet hourly until improved, then every 4 hours. Maximum 5 days.

NUTRITION

Unless absolutely essential, do not take anti-diarrhea drugs for the first 24 hours and do not eat, either. You must replace fluids and electrolytes, so make up 4 cups of freshly boiled water with a mixture of 8tsp of sugar and 1tsp of salt, and drink the whole amount at least twice a day. After 24 hours use the BRAT diet: ripe Bananas, boiled Rice, Applesauce, and dry whole wheat Toast. Eat little and often for the next 48 hours, then add boiled or baked potatoes, cooked carrots with other mixed vegetables, and an egg. Gradually get back to normal eating, saving all dairy products until last.

To relieve diarrhea, crush four cloves of garlic and stir into a 1lb/450g jar of honey (but not for children under two). Dissolve 2tsp in a tumbler of hot water and sip slowly, repeating three times daily.

AROMATHERAPY

⟶ Roman chamomile *(Chamaemelum nobile)*
⟶ Neroli *(Citrus aurantium)*
⟶ Lavender *(Lavandula angustifolia)*
⟶ Peppermint *(Mentha piperita)*
These oils are antispasmodic and help griping stomach pains. Chamomile is an antallergen, useful if the diarrhea is an allergic reaction. Avoid peppermint if you have a gallbladder or liver problem.
Application Apply gentle abdominal massage.

> **Caution**
> *Avoid medicines that claim to stop diarrhea, as they tend to prolong the illness. Reserve them for occasions when it may be hard to use a toilet frequently, such as while you are traveling.*

below Components of the BRAT diet: Banana, Rice, Applesauce, Toast.

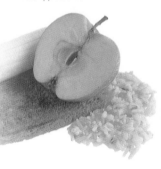

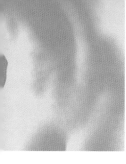

Weight problems

Difficulty in maintaining your weight at the level expected for your height and build; you may weigh either more or less than your ideal weight, or your weight may fluctuate from one to the other; neither extreme of the weight spectrum is healthy.

The **Western world is obsessed with being overweight, but the real truth is that diets often do not work in the long term. At the other end of the scale there are many thousands of people desperate to gain weight. Being severely overweight increases the risk of heart disease, diabetes, respiratory problems, arthritis, and some forms of cancer; being painfully thin increases the risk of osteoporosis, menstrual problems and reduced life expectancy. The overweight will only achieve long-term success by changing the way they eat and increasing their exercise; the overly thin, by eating high-energy foods more frequently.**

🌐 **Call the physician**

If you are seriously concerned about your weight.

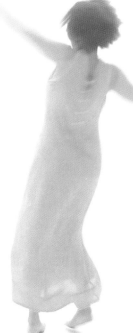

 CONVENTIONAL MEDICINE

To lose weight, eat smaller portions of everything; avoid fatty and sugary food and excessive alcohol. To gain weight, do the reverse, but don't increase your intake of alcohol or sugary food. Regular aerobic exercise produces many health benefits and is essential for healthy weight loss. Treating a serious weight problem may require qualified dietary advice, and in some cases, psychological help.

 HERBAL REMEDIES

Herbal remedies are no real substitute for calorie control, healthy eating and regular exercise, and any proprietary "slimming" tea should be regarded with great suspicion: such teas are usually mixtures of strong laxatives and diuretics, which will have only a short-term effect on weight problems. If the weight problem is associated with a sluggish metabolism or an underactive thyroid, then seeking professional help is generally advisable in such cases. Malabar tamarind is sometimes recommended as a useful treatment for short-term use, as it affects carbohydrate metabolism and can therefore help to prevent overeating.

❊ HOMEOPATHIC REMEDIES

Best treated with a remedy specific to the individual, so consult a qualified homeopath if possible.

 Sulphur 30c

For plump, hearty person with red cheeks. Lazy, untidy, does not feel the cold, and is worse for heat. Very sweaty, with hot feet, put out of bed at night.

Calcarea carbonica 30c

For flabby person, who puts on weight easily. Soft face, pale complexion. Sweaty head at night. Chilly, cold. Cold feet at night in bed and wants to wear socks, removed when feet get too hot.

DOSAGE 1 tablet twice daily. Maximum 1 week.

AROMATHERAPY

People with weight problems often have a very poor self-image, for which frankincense and sandalwood (avoid if you have a kidney problem) oils would be useful. Any citrus or floral oil will help the accompanying depression. Use the oils in a way that supports you—in the bath; in massage; as a perfume; or as a lotion for your face, body, or hands.

🍎 NUTRITION

The only surefire way to lose weight and keep it off is to eat a nutritious, well-balanced diet that is low in fat and calories and high in fiber, and to engage in a program of regular aerobic exercise. So eat plenty of good carbohydrates, such as brown rice, potatoes, whole wheat bread, beans, and pasta; fresh vegetables, fruit, and salads; fish and skinless poultry. Remember: if you have one bad meal, or even a bad week, don't quit; just get yourself back on track as soon as possible.

Those of you desperately trying to gain weight have to increase your calorie consumption without relying on high-fat meat and dairy products. Good carbohydrates (*see above*) are excellent sources of calories, but are bulky. Eat modest amounts of food often, at least every 2–3 hours. Get extra calories from fresh unsalted nuts, seeds, unsalted peanut butter, tahini, avocados, olive oil, and dried fruits.

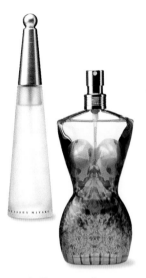

ABOVE Choose a perfume that lifts your mood and improves your self-image.

Caution
Appetite-suppressants are not recommended.

BROWN RICE

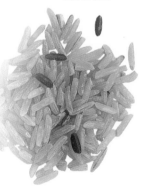

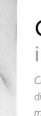

Gastroenteritis,
including food poisoning

Characterized by nausea and vomiting, which may be severe; diarrhea, often quite acute; cramp-like abdominal pain; and mild fever.

cute and violent diarrhea and vomiting may be caused by an infection, but acute gastroenteritis is most commonly caused by food poisoning transmitted by food that has spoiled or been improperly cooked or handled. For an otherwise fit and healthy adult, home remedies can help bring about rapid recovery.

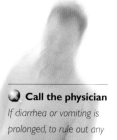

🌀 Call the physician

If diarrhea or vomiting is prolonged, to rule out any underlying illness; if you have been unable to hold down fluids for longer than 12 hours; if there is associated blood or high fever.

➕ CONVENTIONAL MEDICINE

Take a sip of fluid every 5 minutes. If the vomiting continues and symptoms persist for more than 12 hours, seek urgent medical attention. For less severe symptoms, drinking extra water will help, but special oral rehydration fluid preparations are available, tasting like strong mineral water. Prolonged diarrhea may require further treatment, so seek medical advice.

DOSAGE: ADULTS AND CHILDREN Dissolve the contents of an oral rehydration packet in water and drink after each episode of diarrhea; consult label for details.

HERBAL REMEDIES

Herbs can ease the symptoms, while nature gets rid of the irritant.

USE AND DOSAGE Combine a bistort and fenugreek decoction with an agrimony and gotu kola (avoid if pregnant) infusion (1 cup of the mixture, taken three to five times daily) in order to soothe the lower bowel.

Take slippery-elm or marshmallow capsules to protect the gut lining. Bilberry or cranberry juice combats fluid loss while easing bowel discomfort. *Aloe vera* juice is an ideal remedy, if available (avoid if you are pregnant or have a bowel disorder; not for children).

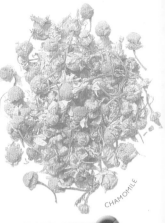

CHAMOMILE

HOMEOPATHIC REMEDIES

Fast for 24 hours, maintaining hydration with sips of water every 15 minutes. The following remedy may be used for travelers' diarrhea.

Arsenicum album 6c

For gastroenteritis from food poisoning. Diarrhea and vomiting at the same time. Chilly, better for warmth. Patient restless, anxious, weak. Heat improves burning abdominal pain. Thirsty for sips of liquid.

DOSAGE 1 tablet hourly until improved, then every 4 hours. Maximum 5 days.

AROMATHERAPY

Roman chamomile (*Chamaemelum nobile*)
Lavender (*Lavandula angustifolia*)
Melissa (*Melissa officinalis*)
Tea tree (*Melaleuca alternifolia*)

Tea tree is antiviral and antibacterial. Chamomile and lavender are soothing and painkilling. Melissa is antidepressant and relieves spasms in the digestive tract.

APPLICATION Tea tree is useful in the home, especially to protect other members of the family—so burn it, and use it to wash all surfaces down, and wash out the bath and any soiled linen. Use the other oils in the bath, in a body lotion, or for massage.

NUTRITION

The first step is always to replace lost fluids and electrolytes (*see Diarrhea on p.98*). You will not feel like eating until the worst symptoms have abated. When you do, avoid all dairy products for at least 48 hours and stick to the BRAT diet—ripe Bananas, boiled Rice, Applesauce, and dry whole wheat Toast (*see p.99*). Do not have any ice-cold drinks and avoid all citrus juices.

Yogurt plays a vital role in recovering from gastroenteritis. Its natural bacteria destroy unwelcome bacteria in the gut and have an immune-boosting effect. This is also true of fermented milk products. Unfortunately, none of these benefits is provided by most commercial yogurts, so you must choose live yogurt, a rich source of beneficial probiotic bacteria.

Caution

Severe gastroenteritis, especially in children or the elderly, may be extremely grave. Avoid medicines that claim to stop diarrhea, as they tend to prolong the illness; reserve them for occasions when it may be hard to use a toilet frequently.

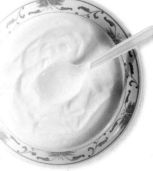

BELOW A portion of live yogurt will soothe the gut and boost the immune system.

Gastritis

Pain or discomfort in the upper abdomen, related to food; may be associated with nausea or belching.

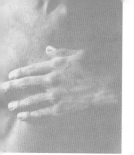

Severe and sudden gastritis—or inflammation of the stomach lining—is nearly always self-inflicted. Too much alcohol, too many cigarettes, very hot curries, and even some medicines can all act as the trigger.

Call the physician
If the symptoms persist or if they are not relieved by antacids.

BELOW A herbal infusion can help to relieve the pain of gastritis.

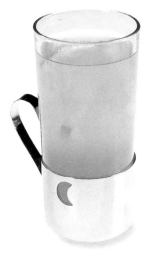

CONVENTIONAL MEDICINE

Avoid NSAIDs, which are often taken for pain-relief. Frequent small meals of bland food may relieve the symptoms. Antacids can also be helpful *(see p.78)*.

HERBAL REMEDIES

USE AND DOSAGE Take slippery elm or marshmallow as tablets or as powders, made into a paste with warm water.

Fenugreek seeds (2tsp per cup) in a decoction with a pinch of powdered cinnamon can bring relief; or use lemon balm, meadowsweet (avoid if you are sensitive to aspirin), and fennel in an infusion (½–1tsp of each per cup). Avoid using cinnamon and fennel if you are pregnant or breastfeeding.

HOMEOPATHIC REMEDIES

Severe or persistent pains, or vomiting blood or dark fluid, require medical attention. A consultation with a qualified homeopath is recommended.

Nux vomica 6c
For gastritis from alcohol. Cannot stand pressure around waist. Cramping pains, worse for eating, anger. Workaholic and irritable.

Capsicum 6c
For burning or icy-cold feeling in stomach. Wants coffee but produces nausea. Lots of flatulence.

DOSAGE 1 tablet taken every 2 hours for six doses, then three times daily. Maximum 3 days.

REPRODUCTIVE
SYSTEM

The Reproductive System

During her lifetime, the average woman will have about 400 menstrual periods, which are regulated by hormones in the bloodstream. Although the hormonal level varies during the cycle, if there is any upset in the balance of the hormones, then menstrual disorders, **PMS**, and menopausal problems may occur. But help is at hand in the form of nutritional supplements, healthy eating, hormone-balancing herbs, destressing oils, and homeopathic remedies.

Menstrual problems

Too frequent, irregular or absent periods (amenorrhea); painful periods (dysmenorrhea); periods that last an exceptionally long time; heavy periods (menorrhagia), possibly with clots.

The menstrual cycle is controlled by your body's production of hormones and anything that interferes with this mechanism—significant loss or gain of weight, stress, anxiety, or depression—will affect your periods. The underlying causes of menstrual disorder may be simple and medically unimportant, or complex and carry serious medical implications, but home remedies can play an important part in resolving many of them. *(See also Osteoporosis on p.70, Menopause on p.110, Fibroids on p.114, and PMS on p.108).*

 CONVENTIONAL MEDICINE

Most changes in the menstrual cycle are transient, but if there has been a sustained change for more than 6 months, your doctor may wish to investigate. Painful periods may be treated with prescription pain relievers containing mefenamic acid (an anti-inflammatory drug), which also helps to reduce the amount of blood flow. Pregnancy is the most common cause of a missed period. Excessive weight loss and exercise can also stop periods.

HOMEOPATHIC REMEDIES

It is useful to consult a qualified homeopath.

Magnesium phosphate 30c

For colicky abdominal pains, eased by hot-water bottle and pressing firmly on abdomen. Better when period is flowing.

Cimicifuga racemosa 30c

For labor-like pains from hip to hip. Worse for movement. Pains worse, the heavier the period. Better for bending double. Person is chilly and thirsty.

Sepia 30c

For cramping, heavy pains in uterus. Better for sitting with crossed legs. Tired.

DOSAGE 1 tablet 2–4 hourly. Maximum 12 doses.

 Call the physician

If you are having long-term or very uncomfortable menstrual problems.

HERBAL REMEDIES

Warming herbal teas help soothe period pain.

Use and Dosage Mix equal amounts of St. John's wort, raspberry leaves, and skullcap (2tsp per cup).

White willow and black haw help relax cramping pains: take 4tsp of the tincture as a single dose in warm water; repeat after 4 hours if necessary.

For heavy periods use a tea of lady's mantle, shepherd's purse, and marigold (2tsp of each per cup).

Chasteberry (vitex) is a hormone regulator: use 20 drops of tincture in water each morning.

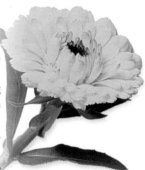

ABOVE Marigold can be combined with shepherd's purse and lady's mantle to relieve heavy periods.

NUTRITION

What you eat and drink plays a vital part in the solution of all menstrual problems. Eat plenty of whole grain cereals, yeast extracts, wheat germ, dried fruits, nuts, bananas, and oats for their vitamin B; oily fish for its essential fatty acids; cold-pressed oils, wheat germ, avocados, and all edible seeds for their vitamin E. Get lots of zinc (from shellfish, sardines, pumpkin seeds, and peas) and selenium (from whole wheat bread, Brazil nuts, almonds, and soy products). Add some borage flowers to salad to help relieve the discomfort of menstrual problems.

If you are constantly dieting, your weight is going down, and your periods are irregular, you may be at risk for anorexia and an artificially induced menopause. Heavy periods increase the risk of iron deficiency and anemia, so eat more of the foods rich in iron: liver (in limited quantities or not at all if you're pregnant), dark green leafy vegetables, raisins, watercress, and eggs.

RAISINS

AROMATHERAPY

🌿 Rose *(Rosa damascena/Rosa centifolia)*
🌿 Geranium *(Pelargonium graveolens)*
🌿 Clary sage *(Salvia sclarea)*

These oils relate to the feminine aspect and help women feel they are in control of their own bodies.

Application Use in the bath, in massage oil or lotion, or as a compress.

Prevention

Try to avoid constipation (see p.96), which can cause pressure on the abdomen and aggravate menstrual problems. So eat plenty of soluble and insoluble fiber (but avoid bran) and drink at least 6pt/2.75liter of liquid each day. An excess of alcohol or caffeine may interfere with blood flow to the uterus and lead to menstrual difficulties, while salt can be a major hazard, since it leads to fluid retention—which is the last thing you need when you are having a period.

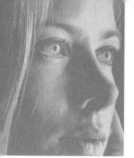

Premenstrual syndrome: PMS

Recurrent symptoms may include back ache, headache, bloated abdomen, cramps, breast tenderness, irrational behavior, anxiety, depression, and poor concentration.

Premenstrual syndrome is the most common of all menstrual problems *(see p.106)*. About **70 percent of women** who are still having a menstrual cycle will suffer from it to some extent. The physical and mental changes may begin just after mid-cycle, but usually occur in the seven days preceding menstruation and vanish as soon as the period starts. Even mild cases of **PMS** can be distressing. Yet, from a medical point of view, it is still a much underrated problem.

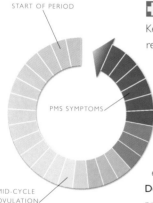

START OF PERIOD

PMS SYMPTOMS

MID-CYCLE OVULATION

ABOVE Monitoring your menstrual cycle enables you to become familiar with potential problems and take remedial steps accordingly.

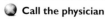

Call the physician

If your symptoms are significantly interfering with your life.

CONVENTIONAL MEDICINE

Keep a chart showing when symptoms occur in relation to menstruation, to enable you to rearrange schedules to avoid particularly difficult days and help to determine whether remedies are of benefit. Breast pain may be helped by products that contain evening primrose oil, an essential fatty acid. If premenstrual syndrome is severe, your physician may recommend hormonal treatments and possibly even counseling.

DOSAGE: WOMEN OVER 16   3–4 capsules of evening primrose oil twice a day, usually for 2–3 months; consult label for details.

HERBAL REMEDIES

Chasteberry (vitex) is often an effective remedy for premenstrual syndrome.

USE AND DOSAGE Take 10–20 drops of tincture each morning, increasing to 20–40 drops in the 10 days before the period is due.

Dong Quai (avoid if pregnant) is also becoming more readily obtainable.

You can make a simple herbal tea from equal amounts of St. John's wort, raspberry leaves, and vervain for daily use.

❖ HOMEOPATHIC REMEDIES

A prescription based on the individual is usually most successful, so consult a qualified homeopath.

☙ **Lilium tigrinum 30c**

For snappy, irritable person. Worse for sympathy. Must keep busy. Heavy period pains, uterus feels as though congested.

☙ **Pulsatilla 30c**

For weepy person, who feels unloved and wants sympathy. PMS starts at puberty. Changeable in mood and symptom. Chilly, but dislikes stuffy room.

DOSAGE I tablet twice daily until improved. Maximum I week. May be repeated at the next period.

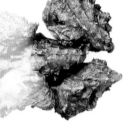

ABOVE Oysters are an excellent source of zinc, which plays a role in regulating PMS.

AROMATHERAPY

☙ Geranium *(Pelargonium graveolens)*
☙ Clary sage *(Salvia sclarea)*
☙ Rose *(Rosa damascena/Rosa centifolia)*
☙ Ylang ylang *(Cananga odorata)*
☙ Neroli *(Citrus aurantium)*
☙ Vetivert *(Vetiveria zizanoides)*
☙ Jasmine *(Jasminum officinale)*
☙ Bergamot *(Citrus bergamia)*

You will have to decide, by a process of trial and error, which of these oils best suits your own range of symptoms. (Do not use jasmine for babies or small children.)

APPLICATION Use in a way that suits your condition.

NUTRITION

It is not just what you eat that is important, but what you *don't* eat and *when* you eat. Women with PMS should eat little and often (never going more than 2 hours without food) and include plenty of complex carbohydrates (whole wheat bread, rice, pasta, potatoes, root vegetables, beans) with sensible protein like fish, eggs, cheese, poultry, and lean meat. Sweet cravings can be satisfied by fruit. Eat plenty of dark green leafy vegetables and whole wheat bread; extra-virgin olive oil, nuts, and seeds; shellfish, oysters, and pumpkin seeds. Avoid consuming excessive salt, caffeine, and alcohol.

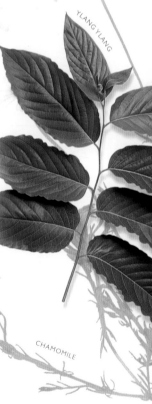

YLANG YLANG

CHAMOMILE

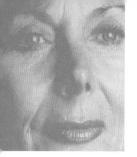

Menopause

No periods for more than one year; sudden attacks of hot flashes; dry vagina, sometimes causing pain during intercourse; urinary problems, including incontinence; may be associated with depression and anxiety.

ome women sail through the menopause; for others, it is a time of misery. But the menopause is not a disease; it is, in fact, for many women, the beginning of years free from the monthly discomfort of difficult periods and contraception. Hormone replacement therapy and home remedies can alleviate symptoms, strengthen bones, protect against heart disease, and keep your skin healthy. Anorexia, overexercising, and being too thin can all affect hormone production and cause an artificial menopause. Removal of both ovaries has the same result.

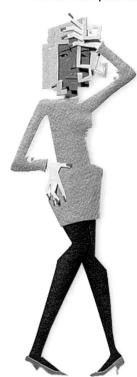

ABOVE Symptoms of the menopause can be controlled to let you lead a full and active life.

 CONVENTIONAL MEDICINE

Hormone replacement therapy (HRT) can help to alleviate difficult symptoms and to reduce the risk of osteoporosis and heart disease in later life. It is given in the form of tablets, patches, gels, or cream, and may cause a regular monthly period. Consult your physician for further details.

HERBAL REMEDIES

Night sweats, hot flashes, and palpitations may be eased by herbal remedies.

USE AND DOSAGE Make up equal amounts of black cohosh, vervain, sage, mugwort, and motherwort (2tsp per cup) as a tea. Sage is rich in hormonal compounds, so a daily cup can be helpful, but avoid if pregnant. The Chinese herbal tonic for this time of life is He Shou Wu (also called Fo Ti), but do not use if you have phlegm or diarrhea.

 AROMATHERAPY

- Geranium *(Pelargonium graveolens)*
- Rose *(Rosa damascena/Rosa centifolia)*
- Fennel *(Foeniculum vulgare)*

Geranium helps to balance the hormones; fennel produces a plant estrogen (avoid if pregnant); and rose regulates the menstrual cycle. Also try any of the antidepressant oils or those for symptomatic conditions, such as constipation (see p.96).

APPLICATION Use in baths, in creams, or in foot spas—whatever method is most convenient for you. Supplementation with starflower may also help.

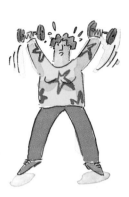

✿ HOMEOPATHIC REMEDIES

Homeopathy can be used to treat the symptoms of the menopause.

☙ Lachesis 30c

For person who may be talkative, jealous, worse for any sleep or alcohol. Palpitations and flushes. Probably the remedy used most often.

☙ Sepia 30c

For lack of emotions, indifference to own family, loss of sex drive. Weeping and feelings of guilt. Flushes with fainting. Better for being alone.

DOSAGE I tablet twice daily. Maximum I week.

⬛ NUTRITION

Good nutrition is the easiest way to reduce the risk of post-menopausal complications, especially if you decide not to take HRT. Plan your daily eating to include the specific nutrients your body now needs in greater abundance than ever. For calcium and vitamin D to protect your bones, eat plenty of low-fat dairy products, sardines and other oily fish (with their bones when possible), dark green leafy vegetables, and chickpeas. For vitamins A, C, and E, beta-carotene, soluble fiber, and essential fatty acids, eat avocados, olive oil, nuts and seeds, oats, brown rice, whole grain cereals, apricots, carrots, and broccoli, liver at least once a week, and lots of oily fish. Especially beneficial are cabbage and its relatives and soybean products; eat these foods often.

This is one time in your life when regular vitamin and mineral supplements can be a real bonus: a daily multivitamin and mineral supplement, a calcium with vitamin D supplement, and Ig of evening primrose oil. To help with hot flashes, a combination of vitamin B_6, magnesium, and zinc can be added.

BELOW Curly kale is full of vitamin D, essential for strong bones.

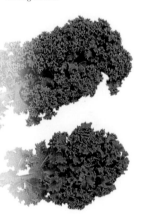

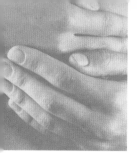

Yeast infections

*Symptoms are a thick, creamy-white vaginal discharge;
sore, itchy vagina, with discomfort along the lips of the
vagina; painful intercourse; and a burning sensation when
passing urine.*

aginal yeast infections are caused by the fungus Candida *albicans,*
one of several species of fungi that normally grow in the vagina.
(Candida **infections can also affect the anus and the mouth.) Vaginal
yeast infections occur when weakened resistance or antibiotic treatments, among other factors, upset the normal bacterial balance of the
vagina, allowing** Candida albicans **to proliferate abnormally. For many
years, the home remedies of complementary practitioners have
offered effective treatment for this common but irritating condition.**

 CONVENTIONAL MEDICINE

Conventional treatment usually consists of antifungal
medications, which can either be inserted into the
vagina as a cream or suppository or taken by mouth
as a single tablet. When a woman has recurrent vaginal yeast infections, her partner may also need to
have treatment.

DOSAGE: ADULTS Follow medical advice on the use
of either creams or suppositories. Alternatively, a
single tablet can be taken by mouth. All treatment
may be combined with an antifungal cream for
external use.

BELOW Lemon balm is
antifungal and can be
beneficial for those with
yeast infections.

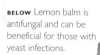

HERBAL REMEDIES

Antifungal and antiseptic herbs—such as echinacea
(avoid if you are pregnant or have a disorder of the
immune system), garlic, chamomile, lemon balm,
thyme, and marigold—as well as immune stimulants
like astragalus and reishi (avoid if pregnant) can help.
USE AND DOSAGE Try an infusion of marigold, lemon
balm, chamomile, and elderflowers (2tsp per cup,
four times daily).

Also try tea-tree, garlic clove, or thyme oil pes-
saries, or put 2 drops of tea-tree oil on a moistened
tampon, insert and leave for up to 4 hours.

HOMEOPATHIC REMEDIES

A consultation with a homeopath is recommended.

Borax 6c

For itchy vulva. Discharge thick or like white of egg, makes vulva sore. Discharge before and after period.

Helonias 6c

For creamy-white discharge, which may recur with itching and soreness of vulva.

DOSAGE 1 tablet twice daily. Maximum 2 weeks.

Candida albicans 30c

For recurrent yeast infections.

DOSAGE 1 tablet twice a day. Maximum three doses.

 AROMATHERAPY

Lavender *(Lavandula angustifolia)*
Tea tree *(Melaleuca alternifolia)*
Myrrh *(Commiphora molmol)*
Palmarosa *(Cymbopogon martinii)*

Lavender eases the pain and promotes healing. Tea tree and myrrh act against the organism that causes yeast infections (but use tea tree in a low dilution, as it can irritate the mucous membrane). Palmarosa helps to balance intestinal flora. Treatment needs to be long-term or infection may recur.

APPLICATION Use in the bath or as a compress on the outer areas. Palmarosa can also be used as a massage oil for the abdominal area.

 NUTRITION

Garlic is a powerful antifungal and should be used generously—eat at least 2 whole cloves a day. It also helps to eat a good portion of live yogurt daily, to maintain the balance of beneficial probiotic bacteria in the gut, which may help prevent the spread of the *Candida* infection. All the B vitamins are important too, so eat plenty of complex carbohydrates, like whole wheat pasta and brown rice, as well as extra muesli, sunflower seeds, lentils, and white fish for their rich vitamin B_6 content. Get extra zinc from eggs, sardines, oysters, other shellfish, and pumpkin seeds. On the other hand, avoid dietary sources of yeast, such as bread and beer.

Prevention

Avoid wearing synthetic panties, and make sure pantyhose have a cotton gusset—or, better still, wear stockings. Avoid very hot baths, antiseptic soaps, excessive washing, and all highly perfumed, foaming bath additives.

Some complementary practitioners advise extreme yeast-excluding diets, but there is no scientific evidence of their effectiveness. It is advisable, however, to reduce your sugar consumption, since a high sugar intake can promote the growth of Candida.

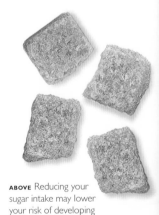

ABOVE Reducing your sugar intake may lower your risk of developing yeast infections.

CRAMP
BARK

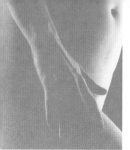

Fibroids

Most women have no symptoms, but there may be heavy menstrual bleeding; an urge to pass urine frequently, caused by the fibroids pressing on the bladder; swelling in the lower part of the abdomen.

About 20 percent of women over the age of 35 will develop fibroids, benign tumors that grow in the smooth muscle of the uterus. More prevalent among women of African descent, fibroids are probably the most common reason for a hysterectomy, although less invasive medical techniques are now available for removing them. Self-help methods may contain fibroid growth until menopause, when reduced estrogen levels cause a gradual reduction in fibroid size.

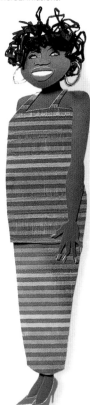

BELOW Women with fibroids may benefit from drinking simple herbal infusions.

CONVENTIONAL MEDICINE

Most fibroids do not need any treatment, but if symptoms are troublesome, seek medical advice. If medicines are unsuccessful, surgery may remove the fibroids or the whole uterus (hysterectomy).

HERBAL REMEDIES

Treatment should really be left to professionals, although simple remedies can ease symptoms.
USE AND DOSAGE Cramp bark or black haw, in decoction or tinctures, eases pain. Shepherd's purse infusion (1tsp per cup) can help stop bleeding. Or make a tea of violet leaves, shepherd's purse and motherwort (2tsp per cup, drunk three times a day).

HOMEOPATHIC REMEDIES

It is best to consult a qualified homeopath. The following remedies may be a guide.

Ustilago 6c
For left-sided ovarian pain, which may extend to the legs. Fibroids with heavy periods and clots, especially when approaching the menopause.

Fraxinus americana 6c
For fibroids with heavy feeling in vagina. Watery vaginal discharge.
DOSAGE 1 tablet daily. Maximum 2 weeks.

The Excretory System

The kidneys filter about 300pt/150liter of fluid each day, producing about 1⅞pt/900ml of urine and returning the rest to the circulation. If the bladder or urethra becomes infected, cystitis may result; bedwetting, on the other hand, may occur for no apparent reason and is usually self-limiting in children. Piles or hemorrhoids are another uncomfortable disorder of the excretory system. But simple nutritional, aromatherapeutic, herbal, and homeopathic remedies, supported by conventional treatment, can provide effective relief for all these ailments.

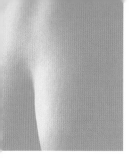

Hemorrhoids

Characterized by bleeding, often a bright red streak on the bathroom tissue or surface of the feces; part of the bowel may prolapse (stick out) when feces are passed, then may return or stay out.

I **f you have had children, suffer from constipation, stand a lot at work, or are seriously overweight, the chances are that you will suffer from hemorrhoids (or piles, as they are more colloquially known) at some point. If severe, hemorrhoids—which are varicose veins in the soft lining of the anus—may require surgical treatment, but home remedies can provide great relief for most people.**

Call the physician

If you have had any bleeding from the anus, in order to rule out a more serious cause.

CONVENTIONAL MEDICINE

Eat plenty of high-fiber foods, such as apples, pears, beans, oats, whole wheat bread, and brown rice. Drink plenty of water. This will help to keep the feces soft and easier to pass without straining. Your physician may prescribe suppositories together with a cream containing anti-inflammatory drugs.

HERBAL REMEDIES

One traditional herb for hemorrhoids is witch hazel. It is astringent and cooling, and relieves the itching caused by hemorrhoids.

USE AND DOSAGE Make a compress with witch hazel whenever you need relief.

Infusions of yarrow, lime flowers, or sweet clover will help the circulation and blood vessels. Other possible remedies are fresh *Aloe vera* leaves, chickweed cream, or borage juice, which can also help to relieve itching. Avoid sweet clover, however, if you are pregnant.

HOMEOPATHIC REMEDIES

Unexplained or persistent rectal bleeding requires medical attention. Paeonia ointment may help to relieve the itching.

 Aesculus 6c

For sensation of splinters felt in rectum. Pain

extends to hips. Large, painful and protruding, purple hemorrhoids. Anus is dry and itchy.

🕭 **Aloe 6c**

For hemorrhoids like bunches of grapes. Purple color, better for cold bathing. Itching in rectum.

🕭 **Hamamelis 6c**

For hemorrhoids in pregnancy, profuse bleeding with soreness.

Dosage: 1 tablet twice daily. Maximum 2 weeks.

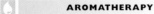

AROMATHERAPY

🕭 **Cypress** *(Cupressus sempervirens)*
🕭 **Geranium** *(Pelargonium graveolens)*
🕭 **Juniper** *(Juniperus communis)*
🕭 **Myrrh** *(Commiphora molmol)*

Cypress is a natural astringent, which can help shrink the piles. Avoid cypress and juniper if you are pregnant and juniper if you have a kidney problem.

APPLICATION Use either alternate hot and cold sitz baths or 3–4 drops of your chosen oil in a warm compress, held on the anus or against the hemorrhoid. Or add about 10 drops of geranium and 10 drops of cypress to a tube of lubrication jelly.

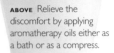

ABOVE Relieve the discomfort by applying aromatherapy oils either as a bath or as a compress.

NUTRITION

During an episode of painful hemorrhoids, it is important to keep the stool as soft as possible. Dried fruits, especially prunes and apricots, and a regular intake of prune juice will help. Avoid the temptation not to pass stools, however painful it might be, as further constipation will only make the piles worse. Plenty of fluid and foods rich in soluble fiber, such as oats, apples, pears, and nearly all vegetables, will help prevent constipation leading to hemorrhoids. If you are constantly losing even small amounts of blood from your piles there is a risk of anemia, so take nutritional steps to prevent this *(see p.56)*. This is particularly important for women, especially during pregnancy.

Avoid food with lots of seeds (e.g. tomatoes, raspberries) until your condition has settled down, because these can cause further irritation.

Caution

Do not apply the essential oils undiluted. If there is any bleeding, seek medical advice before using essential oils.

Prevention

Exercise regularly. Avoid prolonged sitting or standing, and straining during bowel movements. To stimulate blood flow to the rectum, take daily hot/cold water contrast baths.

Cystitis

Painful, burning sensation when passing urine, often worse at end of stream; urine may be pink, due to the presence of blood; there may be small blood clots; frequent need to go to the bathroom, perhaps only passing a small amount; fever.

ystitis can be an isolated acute problem or a recurring chronic nightmare, which affects millions of women but few men. It is often impossible to trace the specific bacteria that trigger an episode of cystitis, which is often linked to concurrent yeast infections *(see p.112)*. Recurrent episodes may be treated with prophylactic antibiotics.

🌐 Call the physician

If you have a high fever with cystitis and/or vomiting; if you have cystitis with back pain; if your symptoms persist.

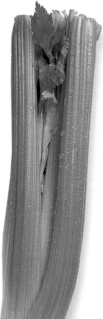

BELOW Celery and other diuretic foods will help flush out the system.

✚ CONVENTIONAL MEDICINE

"Over-the-counter" remedies help neutralize the acid in the urine. If symptoms remain, antibiotics are usually required to prevent the infection from spreading to the kidneys.

DOSAGE: ADULTS Take antibiotics as directed; follow medical advice.

DOSAGE: CHILDREN Seek medical advice. Dose depends on the age and weight of the child; follow medical advice and remember to complete the whole course.

▢ NUTRITION

Drink at least 8–10 glasses of water each day, and make sure you eat lots of diuretic foods, such as celery. Avoid caffeine, drink little alcohol and only weak tea.

The traditional kitchen treatment for cystitis is lemon barley water. Pour 7 cups of boiling water over ¼ cup of washed barley and the grated rind and juice of an unwaxed lemon. Add ½tsp of sugar, stir thoroughly, and drink one glass three times a day. Modern scientific research, however, has now proved that a traditional Native American remedy—cranberry juice—is even more effective. Chemicals in the juice seem to prevent the cystitis-causing bacteria from making their home in the bladder tissue. Drink at least 2–3 glasses a day of a

50:50 dilution of cranberry juice with water. This acts both as treatment during an attack of cystitis and as long-term protection.

HERBAL REMEDIES

Many herbs act as urinary antiseptics and can be helpful in combating infections and inflammation, while drinking herbal teas increases fluid intake.

USE AND DOSAGE Take up to 4 cups daily of a tea made from 1 part each of buchu, couchgrass, and bearberry (2tsp per cup of water). Add 2 parts shepherd's purse if there is blood in the urine, but make sure that you seek professional advice if symptoms persist. Do not use if you are pregnant or have kidney problems.

Avoid spicy foods and those producing acid residues, such as meat and shellfish.

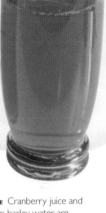
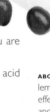

ABOVE Cranberry juice and lemon barley water are effective in the treatment and prevention of cystitis.

AROMATHERAPY

- Myrrh *(Commiphora molmol)*
- Tea tree *(Melaleuca alternifolia)*
- Roman chamomile *(Chamaemelum nobile)*
- Lavender *(Lavandula angustifolia)*

These oils are calming, soothing, and anti-inflammatory; tea tree is antiviral, antifungal, and antibacterial.

APPLICATION Use in a warm compress over the lower back, in sitz baths or in ordinary baths.

HOMEOPATHIC REMEDIES

Symptoms in males or worsening symptoms, back pain, or chills require medical help.

- **Cantharis 30c**

For "peeing red hot needles." Constantly wanting to urinate, but passing just a few drops. Urine may be bloody.

- **Staphysagria 30c**

For "honeymoon cystitis." Burning pain after intercourse or after having had a catheter inserted. Recurrent cystitis related to intercourse.

DOSAGE 1 tablet every 4 hours until condition improves. Maximum 5 days.

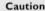

Caution

If blood or pus appears in the urine, contact your physician immediately.
If antibiotics are prescribed, continue with the aromatherapy treatment, as they will work side-by-side.

Bedwetting: enuresis

Uncontrollable urge to pass urine in a child who is learning to use a toilet; adults may also suffer, particularly after undergoing an alcoholic binge.

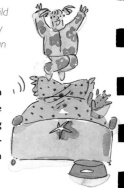

edwetting is much more common in boys than girls, and most children grow out of it by the age of four or five. It is seldom the result of underlying disease, although occasionally it may be. Stress, anxiety, or other behavioral disturbances can result in bedwetting, but in most instances, it "just happens."

 Call the physician
If bedwetting does not improve after trying these remedies.

BELOW With very young children, patience and understanding might be the only treatment that is needed.

 CONVENTIONAL MEDICINE

There is no fixed age at which a child should be dry at night, but bedwetting from the age of seven is often treated by physicians with medication. A child who has been dry might wet the bed when starting a new school, or because of a urine infection. Avoid scolding or withholding drinks—encouragement to use the toilet is more effective. Reward a dry night.

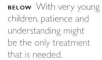 **HERBAL REMEDIES**

During the day, give dilute herbal teas to help strengthen the bladder and soothe distress.
USE AND DOSAGE Mix 1tsp each of cornsilk, shepherd's purse, and skullcap and infuse in 1 cup/250ml of water. Give children under three half a cup (with a teaspoon of sugar, if necessary), two to three times daily. One hour before bedtime give 10 drops of sweet sumach tincture, diluted in 1tsp of water.

 HOMEOPATHIC REMEDIES

✿ **Causticum 6c**
For sensitive person, who wets bed during early part of sleep or in daytime when sneezing/coughing.
✿ **Equisetum 6c**
For person who has dreams/nightmares when passing urine. Bedwetting in children and elderly women.
DOSAGE 1 tablet before bed. Maximum 2 weeks.

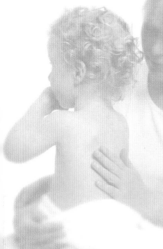
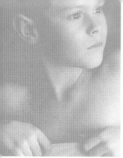

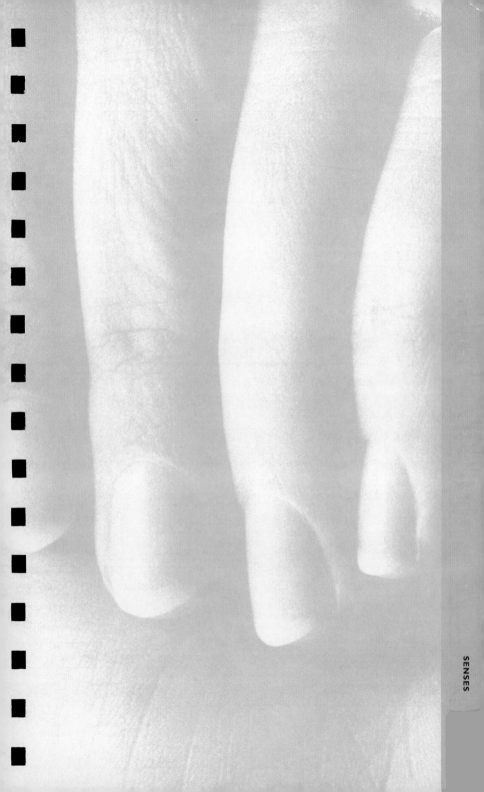

The Senses

The largest organ of our bodies, skin is a remarkable material, serving as a protective barrier for all the internal body organs, eliminating waste products through sweat, and ultrasensitive to pain, touch, and temperature. But it is also subject to numerous disorders, from acne and warts to dermatitis and cellulite, and needs nourishment in order to remain healthy. The other sense organs—ears, eyes, and mouth and tongue—are also subject to a variety of problems such as earache, conjunctivitis, and mouth ulcers. But relief is available through both internal and external remedies.

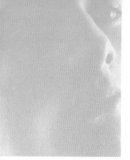

Acne

*Characterized by oily skin, blackheads, and pimples, most
frequently appearing on the face, but also sometimes
erupting on the neck, shoulders, back, or chest; most common
among teenagers.*

Acne is a distressing skin problem that affects around 80 percent of
young people between the ages of 12 and 24. It occurs as a result
of a buildup of oil or sebum secreted through the pores, which become
blocked, then infected, causing pimples. It is more common in boys
than girls and is triggered by the fluctuating levels of hormones during
adolescence. Diet can play a vital part in improving, or worsening, acne.

✚ CONVENTIONAL MEDICINE

Mild acne may only require a lotion that dries the
skin. In moderately severe cases, an antibiotic
preparation applied to the skin may be used in
combination with a drying lotion. If acne is persistent, antibiotics may be effective. In severe cases,
treatment with a derivative of vitamin A may be
prescribed by a dermatologist. Most treatments
take up to 3–6 months to work and may need to
be continued beyond this.

BELOW Teenagers should
eat a diet high in fruit and
vegetables to keep their
system as free as possible
from the toxins that
encourage acne.

DOSAGE: ADULTS AND CHILDREN Apply lotions
and creams to the whole area, not just the
blemishes, twice a day. Take tablets once a
day or more often; follow medical advice.

◻ HERBAL REMEDIES

Combine cleansing herbs taken internally with
external antiseptic washes, steam baths, or lotions.
USE AND DOSAGE Drink 3 cups daily of a tea made
by infusing ⅓oz/10g each of agrimony, burdock leaves, and marigold petals in 1pt/500ml
of water.

Apply a lotion of 4tbsp each of distilled
witch hazel and rosewater with 1tsp each
of tea-tree and thyme oils.

You can also rub acne pustules with a
garlic clove each night.

AROMATHERAPY

- Lavender *(Lavandula angustifolia)*
- Bergamot *(Citrus bergamia)*
- Tea tree *(Melaleuca alternifolia)*

These oils are bactericidal and relaxing, which will help with stress. Tea tree builds up the body's immune system.

APPLICATION Apply undiluted lavender with a cotton ball directly to the blemish. All three oils can be used in a compress or facial steamer; and in a bath.

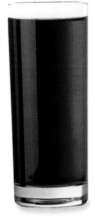

ABOVE Sweet, carbonated drinks and chocolate should be avoided if a clear skin is to be maintained.

NUTRITION

Avoid high-fat, high-sugar convenience foods; eliminate chocolate, ice cream, salt, burgers, and all manufactured meat products. A detox program of raw fruit, vegetables, and salads with unlimited water, unsalted vegetable juices, and herbal teas should be followed for 3 days each month. After the third day add whole grains and cooked vegetables, returning to your normal diet on the fourth day.

Eat plenty of dark green and orange vegetables and fruit for their beta-carotene; citrus fruits for their vitamin C; tropical fruits for their high enzyme content; nuts, seeds, and vegetable oils for their vitamin E. Eat some cabbage every day. Complex carbohydrates, like potatoes, brown rice, and whole wheat bread, can be eaten in abundance. Use vegetarian protein sources or fish and lean poultry.

Caution

Do not apply any oil other than lavender directly to the skin.

KIWI FRUIT

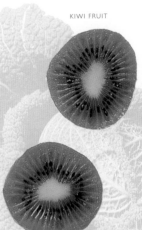

HOMEOPATHIC REMEDIES

A consultation with a homeopath is recommended.

- Kali bromatum 6c

For acne of face, cheek, and forehead. Pimples look bluish-red, discharge pus, and produce scars.

- Sulphur 6c

For pimples on forehead and nose. Skin worse for washing, sensitive to cold air. Pimples that are scratched discharge pus. Patient intolerant of heat, lazy, and produces smelly sweat.

DOSAGE I tablet daily. Maximum 2 weeks.

Boils

*An infection that starts around a hair follicle, forming pus,
with localized swelling; hot, red skin over the affected area;
pain, often throbbing, sometimes associated with a yellow
discharge of pus.*

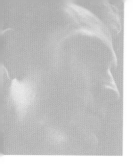

Anyone can get a boil at any time. The occasional episode is
painful and unpleasant, but not of great significance, as long as it
is treated correctly. Repeated boils may, however, be a sign of underlying illness (for example, diabetes) or an indication that your natural
resistance has declined for some reason. The most likely sites for boils
to erupt are at the back of the neck, on the nostrils, armpits, and
between the legs and buttocks.

BELOW A boil is unsightly
and depressing, but it
seldom has any long-
term effects.

 CONVENTIONAL MEDICINE

A boil may burst spontaneously or it may need
lancing in order to release the pus. Treatment at an
early stage with antibiotics can sometimes prevent
a boil from developing, as can cleaning all cuts well
with soap and water.

DOSAGE: ADULTS Take a complete course of
antibiotics as prescribed by your physician;
follow medical advice.

DOSAGE: CHILDREN See your physician; follow
medical advice.

 HERBAL REMEDIES

Traditionally, herbalists have used poultices to
encourage boils to discharge. You can apply commercially available slippery elm or chickweed
ointments, or make a slippery elm poultice yourself.
USE AND DOSAGE Mix 1tsp of powdered slippery
elm with enough hot water, or hot marigold infusion, to make a thick paste, then apply to the boil.
Apply a little echinacea or marigold cream to clear
any remaining infection.

Internally, garlic or echinacea (2 × 200mg capsules, twice a day) will improve resistance to further
infection. Avoid echinacea if you are pregnant or
have a disorder of the immune system.

AROMATHERAPY

∽ Tea tree *(Melaleuca alternifolia)*
∽ Lavender *(Lavandula angustifolia)*
∽ Bergamot *(Citrus bergamia)*
∽ Juniper *(Juniperus communis)*

Lavender is soothing and a natural painkiller, as is bergamot. Juniper helps to detoxify the system, but avoid if you are pregnant or have a kidney problem.
APPLICATION Use tea tree, lavender, and bergamot in a hot compress; juniper and lavender in the bath.

HOMEOPATHIC REMEDIES

∽ **Belladonna 6c**
For sudden onset, skin painful, red, hot, and throbbing. First stages of boil with little pus formation.

∽ **Hepar sulphuris calcareum 6c**
For splinter-like pains at slightest touch. Brings boil to a head. Patient may be bad-tempered.

∽ **Sulphur 6c**
For crops of boils in different places on the body. One boil finishes as another starts.

DOSAGE I tablet every 4 hours for 2–3 days or until improved.

NUTRITION

Eat plenty of vitamin C-rich food—blackcurrants, blueberries, citrus fruit, kiwis, and fresh fruit juices; liver, carrots, broccoli, and spinach for their vitamin A; pumpkin seeds and shellfish for their zinc; garlic and cabbage for their antibacterial properties. Avoiding high-sugar and high-fat foods substantially reduces the risk of getting boils, so eat less sugar and refined carbohydrates and drink fewer sweetened soft drinks.

Prevention

Eating a healthy diet (see Nutrition) *that includes plenty of fresh fruit and vegetables and a low sugar intake, is the best way to avoid getting boils.*

BELOW Blackcurrants, garlic, broccoli, citrus fruit, pumpkin seeds, and shellfish all contain beneficial nutrients.

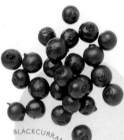

BLACKCURRANTS

GARLIC

BROCCOLI

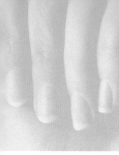

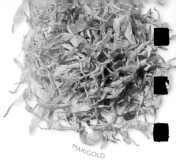

Warts

An unsightly skin growth, often causing no symptoms, although it may be painful if located on the sole of the foot.

MARIGOLD

arts are benign skin growths caused by the human papilloma virus. They occur most often on fingers and the tops of hands, and can spread from one part of the body to another. Common, non-genital warts are usually harmless, although the type that develops on the soles of the feet, called plantar warts, can be quite painful. Ordinary warts are only mildly contagious. Sexually transmitted genital warts, on the other hand, are highly contagious. They are also associated with an increased risk of penile and cervical cancer.

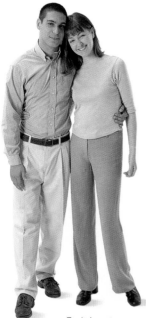

ABOVE Genital warts are very contagious. If one partner develops symptoms, both should seek medical attention.

✚ CONVENTIONAL MEDICINE

Most warts will disappear eventually with no treatment, but because they can spread or, in some cases, cause pain, many people opt to treat them.

The principle of all treatment for warts is to destroy the wart tissue without actually harming the surrounding normal skin. Keep the wart covered to avoid spreading the infection. Before applying a treatment, file the surface of the wart to remove any hard skin, but make sure that the skin is not open or cracked. Seek medical advice for persistent or spreading warts.

DOSAGE: ADULTS AND CHILDREN Apply the treatment daily after filing the surface with an emery board or pumice stone; consult label for details.

HERBAL REMEDIES

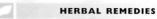

Thuja is extremely antiviral and antifungal.

USE AND DOSAGE A couple of drops of tincture on the wart night and morning will usually clear it reasonably quickly. Also take 5 drops of tincture in a little water twice a day. Avoid if you are pregnant.

Other useful herbs for treating warts include tea-tree oil, marigold, house leeks, and the sap of freshly picked greater celandine.

AROMATHERAPY

ᕗ Lemon *(Citrus limon)*

ᕗ Tea tree *(Melaleuca alternifolia)*

Tea tree is antiviral, while both lemon and tea-tree oil are antiseptic.

APPLICATION Apply undiluted essential oil with a toothpick, so that you get 1 drop directly on the wart. Cover with a dry adhesive bandage and repeat at least twice a day. Alternate the lemon and tea-tree oils after 2 or 3 weeks for maximum effect.

HOMEOPATHIC REMEDIES

ᕗ Thuja 6c

For large, jagged, cauliflower warts. Large, flat warts located on the hands and fingers. Nails deformed. Painful plantar warts. This is probably the most common remedy for warts.

ᕗ Causticum 6c

For warts situated on hands, face and lips. Bleed easily. Warts inflamed and hard; located near or under fingernails.

ᕗ Nitric acid 6c

For large, soft, yellow warts. Especially on eyelids and nose. Bleed on washing. Soft warts.

ᕗ Dulcamara 6c

For smooth, large warts on face or palm.

DOSAGE 1 tablet taken twice daily until improved. Maximum 3 weeks.

NUTRITION

Diet itself cannot really help in treating warts, but foodstuffs have traditionally been used: simple, non-genital warts may respond to rubbing them with the cut end of a clove of garlic or even undiluted lemon juice. Repeat twice daily for a week or two. And if you have a fig tree in your garden, a milky latex can be squeezed from the leaf or stem and dropped onto the wart. Wear rubber gloves and cover the adjacent skin with petroleum jelly. After a few hours an inflamed ring of skin will surround the wart, which should soon shrivel up. Repeat after a few days, if necessary.

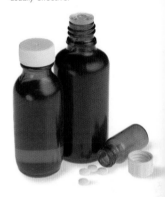

BELOW Treatment with aromatherapy or homeopathic remedies takes several weeks, but is usually effective.

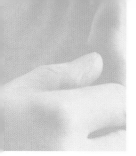

Corns and calluses

*An area of thick, hardened skin, which may be painful;
often found on the toes, although it may also appear on
the hands after rough, repetitive manual work such
as gardening.*

**orns and calluses of the feet are the inevitable result of wearing
ill-fitting shoes. Deformities of the foot can also lead to areas of
excessive pressure or a change of weight distribution when standing or
walking. Either way, corns or calluses may result. Corns should be dealt
with by a physician, qualified podiatrist, or chiropodist and should not be
hacked at with any of the patent corn-removing gadgets. Calluses may
also occur on the palms of the hand and the fingers—for example, as the
result of gardening or manual work.**

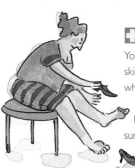

✚ CONVENTIONAL MEDICINE

You can gently file a callus and then moisturize the
skin. It may be easier to file the skin after a bath,
when the skin is soft and pliable.

Covering a corn with a cushioned adhesive
bandage, which is designed to avoid putting pressure directly on the corn itself, can help to relieve
the pain. Otherwise, seek professional advice
from a qualified podiatrist or physician.

❖ HOMEOPATHIC REMEDIES

There are various homeopathic treatments that
may help alleviate corns and calluses.

Antimonium crudum 6c
For thick and distorted nails. Horny lumps on hands
and soles. Callosities from slight pressure. Inflamed
corns. Feet very tender.

Graphites 6c
For thick, ingrown, and crumbling nails. Callosities
on the hands, with skin that cracks and discharges
sticky substance.

Ferrum picricum 6c
For corns with yellowish discoloration. May also be
many warts on the hands.
DOSAGE: 1 tablet twice daily. Maximum 2 weeks.

Prevention
*Shoes should have a round
rather than pointed shape,
and there should be at least
1in/2.5cm between the end of
the longest toe and the tip of
the inside of the shoe. Avoid
high-heeled shoes and pumps,
which cram the foot down
into the toe end.*

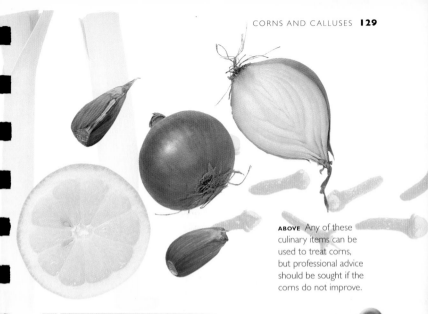

ABOVE Any of these culinary items can be used to treat corns, but professional advice should be sought if the corns do not improve.

HERBAL REMEDIES

There are numerous traditional herbal remedies for corns, such as mashed leeks, onions, garlic cloves, or lemon rind and juice applied directly to the affected area. Inflammation can be soothed with St. John's wort cream or comfrey oil (avoid comfrey if you are pregnant), while easing pressure on the area with thick felt rings. Rubbing the feet with fresh plantain leaves was also believed to prevent corns.

AROMATHERAPY

- Roman chamomile *(Chamaemelum nobile)*
- Lavender *(Lavandula angustifolia)*
- Good-quality vegetable oil (or calendula oil: available from reputable suppliers)

Roman chamomile and lavender are both anti-inflammatory, so they will bring the swelling down and thus lessen the pain of corns and calluses. Using a good-quality vegetable oil will reduce the areas of hardened skin.

APPLICATION Use in a daily massage, especially combining the essential oil with the good-quality vegetable oil. If there is inflammation and the affected area is too tender to touch, then foot baths (or hand baths, if the calluses are on the hand) will be the preferred treatment.

> **Caution**
> *Do not use corn-removing gadgets; instead, seek advice from a qualified podiatrist or chiropodist.*

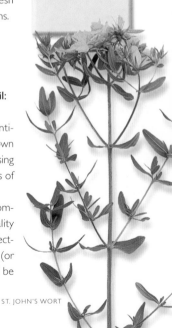

ST. JOHN'S WORT

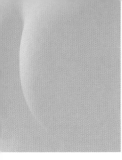

Cellulite

Pitted orange-peel appearance on the skin, most frequently occurring on the upper thighs, buttocks, and arms, where women have a higher proportion of fat than men; primarily a female condition.

This much-discussed and written about "ailment" is not an illness at all. The orange-peel-like skin that characterizes cellulite is not the result of a buildup of toxins, but rather something that happens to the skin of most women—and 98 percent of cellulite sufferers are female. This is because women have a thinner outer skin than men, a thinner underlying level of the dermis, and a different composition of fat cells in the subcutaneous layer. Cellulite is caused by a combination of hormone changes, skin structure, and fat deposits, and though it occurs in women of all sizes, it is more common in those who are overweight.

BELOW A sensible diet is likely to be more effective in reducing cellulite than expensive creams.

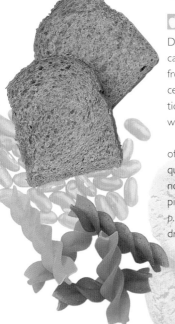

 CONVENTIONAL MEDICINE

Cellulite may improve by taking regular exercise and shedding excess weight, although it tends to worsen during pregnancy. Gently "brushing" the skin each day with a vegetable-bristle brush may help tighten the skin and perhaps reduce cellulite

 NUTRITION

Despite being a cosmetic problem, cellulite is the cause of considerable distress to those suffering from it and, since a woman's total number of fat cells is partially determined by her mother's nutrition during pregnancy, there are certain women who are more prone to it than others.

Weight loss is the first step toward the reduction of cellulite, but do take care: if you lose weight too quickly the condition gets worse. So no crash diets, no ridiculous regimes of meal replacements and pills, just sensible eating *(see Weight Problems on p.100)*, with a reduced intake of refined carbohydrates—from sugars, cookies, cakes, candies, and soft drinks. A diet that is high in complex carbohydrates (such as whole grain cereals, pasta, beans) will ensure that you get an adequate supply of both soluble and insoluble fiber, which in turns helps remove cholesterol from the body. Such a diet also tends to be low in fat. So eat brown rice, oats, beans, whole wheat bread, and pasta for their fiber; bell peppers, broccoli, spinach, and sweet potatoes for their beta-carotene; small amounts of liver for its vitamin A, an essential nutrient for skin health. Reduce your intake of salt and cut down on alcohol, both of which interfere with the efficient circulation of blood to the skin.

> **Caution**
> Rosemary and fennel oils must not be used by those with high blood pressure or epilepsy.

AROMATHERAPY

- Juniper *(Juniperus communis)*
- Fennel *(Foeniculum vulgare)*
- Rosemary *(Rosmarinus officinalis)*

Fennel is a diuretic. Juniper will help the body to detoxify and rosemary helps to stimulate the lymphatic system, which enables the body to remove waste products. If a hormone imbalance is suspected, then geranium could also be used. Do avoid these oils if you are pregnant and avoid juniper if you have a kidney problem.

APPLICATION Use these oils as a massage and in baths (including foot baths). You are looking for long-term benefits, as there is no short-term relief. Remember that stress can be a factor *(see p.36)*.

JUNIPER
BERRIES

HERBAL REMEDIES

Popular demand has created a variety of "over-the-counter" herbal products purporting to reduce cellulite. Most are based on metabolic stimulants, such as kelp, to encourage weight loss and should be avoided. Over-the-counter cellulite remedies based on powerful laxatives (for example, senna, cascara sagrada, rhubarb root), designed to cause sudden weight loss should also be avoided. Patent skin rubs are often based on rubefacient oils, such as juniper, which increase surface blood flow; avoid if you are pregnant or have a kidney problem.

Dermatitis

Starts as a patch of itchy skin covered with small blisters, often after prolonged contact with a mild irritant (such as some soaps and detergents); the area may become raw if it is scratched.

Dermatitis is often an allergic reaction of the skin, producing an acute local inflammation. This may be caused by contact with irritant substances, such as metals, perfumes, cosmetics, or even plants, or it may be part of a general allergic or "atopic" condition, often linked with asthma *(see p.52)* and hay fever *(see p.48)*. Dermatitis caused by direct contact can spread to distant parts of the body. Self-help and simple home remedies can be very effective.

🌐 Call the physician
If the dermatitis is weeping and crusting, since it may be infected.

✚ CONVENTIONAL MEDICINE

Moisturize your skin regularly. If the dermatitis is severe, consult a physician, as treatment with steroid creams may be necessary.

DOSAGE: ADULTS AND CHILDREN Choose a non-perfumed moisturizer; apply as often as possible.

🍎 NUTRITION

Many forms of dermatitis are triggered by foods: both by their natural constituents and by artificial food additives. Handling foods such as garlic, raw fish, and mangoes is another common trigger. Avoiding all artificial additives is the first step toward healing. Then keep a food diary, noting when your skin looks better or worse. The most common irritant foods (in descending order) are milk and all dairy products, shellfish, eggs, citrus fruits, strawberries, red meat, and wheat products.

A high intake of vitamins A and E, beta-carotene, and essential fatty acids is very important, so drink a large glass of carrot juice every day. Eat plenty of broccoli, spinach, tomatoes, apricots, sunflower seeds and oil, oily fish, nuts, soy products, red and green bell peppers, oats, wheat germ, and brown rice. Drink copious amounts of water and eat and celery to stimulate the kidneys.

HOMEOPATHIC REMEDIES

➥ **Kali arsenicosum 6c**

For itching that is intolerable. Worse for warmth, at night, and for undressing. Skin dry and scaly.

➥ **Kreosotum 6c**

For dermatitis on hands and backs of fingers, face, and eyelids. Very itchy. Worse in evening. Better for warmth.

➥ **Petroleum 6c**

For dry, leathery, rough skin with cracks. Burning and itching. Skin may be red, raw, and bleed. Worse in winter.

DOSAGE 1 tablet daily. Maximum 2 weeks (see also Eczema on p.134).

 AROMATHERAPY

➥ **Tea tree** (Melaleuca alternifolia)

➥ **Lavender** (Lavandula angustifolia)

➥ **Roman chamomile** (Chamaemelum nobile)

Tea tree is antiviral, antifungal, and antibacterial. Lavender and chamomile are soothing, anti-inflammatory, and painkilling.

APPLICATION Use in a bath and as a topical cream on the skin. Tea tree can also be used in the washing of towels and facecloths to stop the spread of the infection; make sure the sufferer has separate items from the rest of the family. (See also Eczema on p.134 and Stress on p.36.)

HERBAL REMEDIES

Borage and other herbs are useful in soothing the irritant rash of contact dermatitis.

USE AND DOSAGE Use a lotion made from equal amounts of borage juice and distilled witch hazel. You can make fresh borage juice by pulping the leaves in a food processor; it is also, however, available commercially.

Evening primrose, calendula, or comfrey creams can also help in soothing dermatitis; or you can apply the sap from a fresh Aloe vera leaf to the affected area. Avoid using comfrey if you are pregnant.

Prevention

For contact dermatitis, avoid skin contact with nickel and metal alloys; perfumes, soaps, detergents, and cosmetics are common causes, so buy hypoallergenic varieties. And avoid hair dyes, rubber gloves, many medicated creams and ointments, and some plants, such as primulas, euphorbias, and rue, if you are susceptible. Regular moisturizing of the skin is the most vital part of your daily routine.

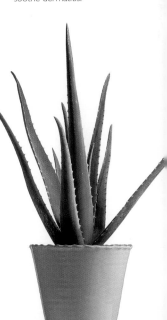

BELOW Aloe vera has many herbal uses and its sap may soothe dermatitis.

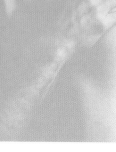

Eczema

Starts with a patch of itchy skin covered with small blisters, which may become red and raw if scratched; in longstanding eczema the skin may become thick, with accentuated markings; sometimes it causes flaky skin—as dandruff on the scalp.

Those unfortunate people who suffer from asthma, hay fever, and eczema are described as atopic. They may have to endure all these problems, and frequently pass them on to their children. There are many similarities between eczema and dermatitis (see p.132) and some conditions labeled dermatitis are in fact eczema.

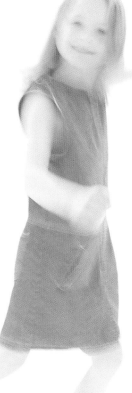

CONVENTIONAL MEDICINE

Moisturize the skin regularly using bath oil, soap substitute, or lotion. If eczema is severe, consult a physician, you may need treatment with steroid creams.
DOSAGE: ADULTS AND CHILDREN Choose a non-perfumed moisturizer; apply as often as possible.

HOMEOPATHIC REMEDIES

Consultation with a homeopath is essential.

Arsenicum album 6c
For dry, rough, scaly skin. Itching and burning. Scratching until skin is raw briefly alleviates this.

Graphites 6c
For rawness in bends of elbows and knees, and behind ears. Oozes pale fluid. Corners of mouth crack. Skin dry and hard.

Sulphur 6c
For dry, burning, scaly skin. Scalp dry. Itching worse for scratching and water.
DOSAGE 1 tablet twice daily. Stop after 2 weeks or on improvement. Repeat if necessary.

NUTRITION

 Call the physician
If the eczema is weeping and crusting, as it may be infected.

Food is frequently a major factor in controlling the flare-up of symptoms, but is not a cure. In asthmatic children, one of the most common culprits is chemical additives—colorings, flavorings, preservatives, and flavor enhancers—which should be avoided.

Early exposure to cow's milk is often the original cause of infantile eczema, so try to avoid giving cow's milk to babies for as long as possible.

All dairy products and citrus fruits can make eczema flare up, but the offending food is often very personal to the individual—from shellfish to strawberries, chocolate to cashew nuts. Compiling a food diary, and noting when the condition becomes better or worse, can help identify the trigger foods; but unless these are few and not essential nutritionally, long-term exclusion diets should be undertaken only under professional guidance.

ABOVE Candies are often high in colorings, preservatives, and other additives.

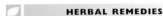

HERBAL REMEDIES

Herbalists generally treat atopic eczema with cleansing herbal teas and limited use of creams.

USE AND DOSAGE Mix equal amounts of red clover, heartsease, burdock leaves, fumitory, and stinging nettles, which will help to reduce inflammation, stimulate the digestion and circulation, and clear any toxins. Use 2tsp of the mixture to a cup of boiling water, three times a day. Avoid if you are pregnant or have a heart or kidney condition. Evening primrose used as an external cream or taken internally (2g per day) can also help. Chickweed, marshmallow, and chamomile creams can all be beneficial.

Caution
Do not apply essential oils to broken, weeping skin without first getting professional advice.

BELOW Keep a food diary to determine which foods—like cow's milk—cause eczema to flare up.

AROMATHERAPY

- Lavender (*Lavandula angustifolia*)
- Roman chamomile (*Chamaemelum nobile*)
- Geranium (*Pelargonium graveolens*)
- Juniper (*Juniperus communis*)
- Rose (*Rosa damascena/Rosa centifolia*)
- Cedarwood (*Cedrus atlantica*)

All these oils are soothing and anti-inflammatory. Juniper is also detoxifying, but may make your condition worse before it gets better (avoid altogether if you are pregnant or have a kidney problem).

APPLICATION Mix calendula base oil with the oils, then rub them gently into the affected area. Alter the formula until you find one that helps your condition. Check for allergies (see p.14) and stress (see p.36).

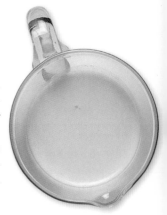

Hives: urticaria

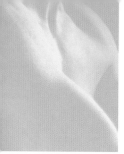

An itchy rash that looks like nettle- or poison-ivy rash, affecting a small area of skin or even the whole body; tends to come and go, leaving no marks, and may improve after a few days or continue for months.

LIPSTICK

Hives—or urticaria, to give it its medical name—is also known as nettle-rash, as its appearance is similar to the lumpy skin eruptions caused by stinging nettles. It is an allergic reaction that can be caused by foods, contact with plants (not necessarily nettles), cosmetics, medications, household cleaning chemicals, alcohol, sudden exposure to cold or hot air, and, very often, by sunlight. Food additives and colorings are frequent culprits, but eruptions of these irritating lumps can also be triggered by stress and anxiety.

BELOW Many foodstuffs are blamed for causing urticaria. Monitor your diet to see which affects you.

 CONVENTIONAL MEDICINE

If you know what triggers the rash, you can avoid it, but in most cases all you can do is try and reduce your symptoms. The rash will be more comfortable if you keep cool. Antihistamines may prevent the rash from developing, although some preparations will make you drowsy. Try calamine lotion to soothe hot, itchy skin.

DOSAGE: ADULTS Most antihistamine tablets are taken once a day; consult label for details, or follow medical advice. Apply calamine lotion/cream directly to the skin as required.

DOSAGE: CHILDREN Doses of antihistamine syrup depend on the age of the child: consult label, or follow medical advice. Apply calamine lotion/cream directly to the skin as required.

NUTRITION

The only long-term treatment is to identify and then avoid the foods that cause attacks by following the exclusion diet *(see p.201)*. The most common irritating foods are shellfish, chocolate, strawberries, eggs, nuts, dairy products, wheat (rarely), and, very commonly, food additives (particularly tartrazine). Aspirin and its derivatives are another common

🌐 **Call the physician**

If the rash persists or if it becomes widespread over the body.

factor in this condition. For those who have identified aspirin as a culprit, it may be worth eliminating all foods that contain natural aspirin as well (most berries, dried and fresh fruit, some nuts and seeds). If your nettle-rash is triggered by sunlight, eat foods rich in beta-carotene: carrots, apricots, spinach, broccoli, bell peppers, and tomatoes. Avoid Earl Grey tea (flavored with bergamot) and buckwheat.

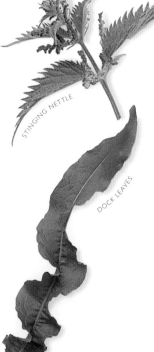

STINGING NETTLE

DOCK LEAVES

AROMATHERAPY

- Roman chamomile *(Chamaemelum nobile)*
- Lavender *(Lavandula angustifolia)*
- Melissa *(Melissa officinalis)*

Chamomile and lavender soothe the irritation; melissa and chamomile calm the allergic reaction.

APPLICATION Use in a light cream base to rub onto the irritated area; in a spray, if the area is too tender to be touched; or in water—either sponge the affected area down or use in the bath.

HOMEOPATHIC REMEDIES

Severe allergic reactions require medical help.

- Urtica urens 30c

For nettle-rash, very itchy red blobs with a white center. Allergic reactions, particularly to shellfish. Worse for cold bathing. Urticaria with joint pains. This is probably the most common remedy.

DOSAGE 1 tablet every 15 minutes until improved. Maximum ten doses.

ABOVE Dock leaves can help to soothe the pain of nettle-rash.

HERBAL REMEDIES

Minor or occasional outbreaks can be soothed with chamomile cream as well as with dock leaves, freshly sliced onion, or crushed cabbage leaves.

USE AND DOSAGE For persistent problems, generally associated with food allergy, make a tea containing agrimony and chamomile (2 parts each) with heartsease and stinging nettles (1 part each), to combat the action of histamine and improve resistance to allergens in the gut. Use 2tsp of the mixture per cup, three times daily. Avoid stinging nettle if you have a heart or kidney condition.

BELOW Crabs and other shellfish are the most common irritating foods.

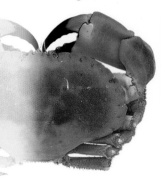

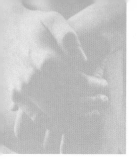

Psoriasis

Thick red patches of skin that are covered by silvery-white scales, often starting on the knees and backs of the elbows, or on the trunk of the body, but sometimes spreading to cover most of the body surface.

Psoriasis is a chronic skin condition, which tends to run in families and affects approximately one person in 50 in both the United States and Britain, although it is much rarer in the black population. It occurs because the skin cells are reproducing far more quickly than normal—the normal cycle takes 311 hours, but in psoriasis it takes just 36. It is more common in smokers and heavy alcohol drinkers, although it can start at any age, most frequently in the late twenties to thirties. Attacks may start with a bacterial throat infection or follow a stressful event; psoriasis can also be a reaction to some drugs.

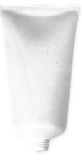

ABOVE Use only non-perfumed moisturizers on affected skin.

 CONVENTIONAL MEDICINE

It is important to keep the skin well moisturized using bath oil, soap substitute, or lotion. Rehumidify the air using a basin of water placed near radiators. If the symptoms persist, seek medical advice—conventional treatment includes prescribed lotions, shampoos, and creams to put on the skin. In more severe cases, treatment with ultraviolet light may help those with psoriasis.

DOSAGE: ADULTS AND CHILDREN Choose a non-perfumed moisturizer; apply as often as possible.

HERBAL REMEDIES

Small areas of psoriasis often respond well to cleavers cream.

USE AND DOSAGE Add 1 cup of strained cleavers infusion to 1 cup of melted emulsifying ointment (available from pharmacies) and stir constantly as it cools and thickens.

Mix equal amounts of the roots of burdock and yellow dock for a decoction (1tsp per cup) or use an infusion of cleavers, red clover flowers, and burdock leaf (2tsp per cup) to alleviate psoriasis. Avoid if you are pregnant.

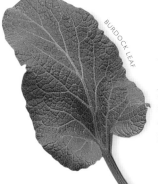

BURDOCK LEAF

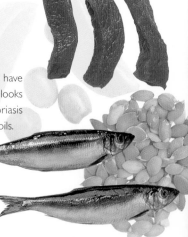

AROMATHERAPY

- Lavender (*Lavandula angustifolia*)
- Basil (*Ocimum basilicum*)
- Bergamot (*Citrus bergamia*)
- Vetivert (*Vetiveria zizanoides*)

The body/mind connection is important: you have psoriasis, so you become stressed because it looks unsightly, and the stress only makes the psoriasis worse. Break the cycle with these destressing oils.

APPLICATION Good base oils are essential—unrefined avocado or carrot oil. Add a few drops of essential oil if you do not want your aqueous cream base to be too greasy. Regular massage from a professional will also help.

HOMEOPATHIC REMEDIES

Consultation with a homeopath is recommended.

- **Sepia 6c**

For itchy psoriasis, not relieved by scratching. On elbows, backs of hands, palms. Scaly, but as soon as one scale comes off another forms.

- **Petroleum 6c**

For dry, cracked, rough skin. Cracked ends of fingers. Worse in winter. Itching at night. Psoriasis on hands.

DOSAGE 1 tablet twice daily. Stop after 2 weeks or on improvement. Repeat if necessary.

ABOVE Orange and red fruit and pumpkin seeds are good for the skin, but some psoriasis sufferers find that fish and red meat worsen their condition.

NUTRITION

Zinc, beta-carotene, vitamin D, and omega-3 fatty acids are essential nutrients. Eat plenty of oily fish for its vitamin D and fatty acids; orange, red and dark green fruit and vegetables for beta-carotene; and shellfish, oysters, and pumpkin seeds for zinc.

Although psoriasis is not an allergic condition, specific foods may aggravate it. Fish, shellfish, citrus fruits, red meat, dairy products, caffeine, and alcohol are the most common triggers. If you notice any of these making your skin worse, try to avoid them. Avoid liver and other organ meat, because they can increase the body's production of normally beneficial complex chemicals, which nonetheless may aggravate psoriasis.

Prevention

There is no specific way to prevent psoriasis, but it is often possible to keep it in check. Sunshine is known to be beneficial, and relaxation techniques may help, for stress is often a major factor. Supplements of vitamin D, beta-carotene, and zinc can also play a part.

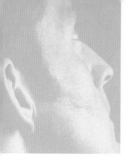

Ringworm: tinea

One or more round areas of scaly, slightly itchy, abnormal-looking skin; the center of the abnormal area may look more normal, leading to the appearance of a ring; usually occurs on moist areas such as the armpits, groin, and feet.

Ringworm is an inflammatory infection of the skin caused by mold or fungi (and 90 percent of all fungal infections are caused by the molds *Microsporum epidermophyton* and *M. trichophyton*). Ringworm infections (so called because of the red patches with a raised outside edge, not because worms are involved), or tinea, thrive in areas of the body that are moist and warm. Home remedies work well in the treatment of this condition. Ringworm is a common and highly contagious infection, spread by direct physical contact. It can be acquired from horses, farmyard animals, and cats *(Microsporum canis)*.

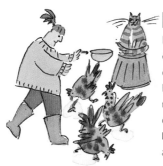

✚ CONVENTIONAL MEDICINE

Ringworm on the body can usually be treated effectively with antifungal creams. If the rash has not cleared up after two weeks, consult your physician. Ringworm that affects the scalp or nails can be more difficult to treat and definitely calls for a discussion with your physician.

DOSAGE: ADULTS AND CHILDREN Most creams are applied twice a day; consult label for details.

❀ HOMEOPATHIC REMEDIES

⤳ Tellurium 6c
For ringworm over whole body, lower limbs. May be more on left side. Itching worse after going to bed, for cool air, and rest. Intersecting rings over whole body.

DOSAGE 1 tablet daily. Maximum 2 weeks.

◗ AROMATHERAPY

⤳ Tea tree *(Melaleuca alternifolia)*
⤳ Myrrh *(Commiphora molmol)*
⤳ Lavender *(Lavandula angustifolia)*
Tea tree and myrrh are antifungal and will attack the fungus that causes ringworm. If lavender is the

only oil you have, you can use this, as it has a slight fungicidal effect.

APPLICATION Apply as a compress; as a water spray (but not too near the eyes); or in a massage medium. Do be aware, however, that ringworm is infectious, and make sure that your hygiene is scrupulous, especially if you are applying oils to somebody else. Wash your hands well afterward, using the oils in the hand wash.

THYME

HERBAL REMEDIES

Tea tree, thyme, and marigold all show antifungal activity and can be very effective for infections such as ringworm.

USE AND DOSAGE Apply tea-tree, thyme, or marigold creams to affected areas three or four times a day.

If the scalp is affected, use a strained marigold infusion as a rinse, or add 5 drops of tea-tree or thyme oil to the rinsing water after shampooing (ideally combined with a strong soapwort infusion, which is very cleansing).

Internally, cleavers and chickweed tea will also help (1 tsp of each per cup).

NUTRITION

Poor nutrition, which results in a lowered natural resistance, can make anyone more susceptible to attack by these ubiquitous molds and fungi. A diet rich in all the essential nutrients, especially vitamins A, C, and E and the minerals zinc and selenium, is generally important for maintenance of the body's natural defenses.

BELOW Raspberries are a rich and delicious source of vitamin C.

So eat plenty of orange and red fruits, dark green leafy vegetables, and liver (in limited quantities or not at all if you are pregnant) for their vitamin A; citrus fruits and other fresh produce for their vitamin C; avocados, nuts, seeds, and olive oil for their vitamin E; shellfish, oysters, and pumpkin seeds for their zinc; and Brazil nuts for their selenium. Regular consumption of garlic acts as a systemic fungicide and is a particularly important remedy if the ringworm has affected the finger- or toenails.

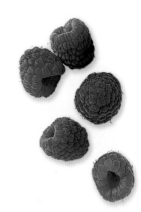

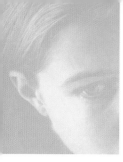

Hair problems

Flaking scalp—likely cause: dandruff; patches of complete hair loss—likely cause: Alopecia areata; *generalized thinning and dry hair—likely cause: underactive thyroid gland; men's hair receding at temples—likely cause: male-pattern baldness.*

air problems are often a sign of underlying illness, as hair is a true barometer of health. Many of the difficulties that arise, however, are simply the result of genetics or of not caring for your hair properly. Most women lose hair after childbirth, but it does grow back again; the same is true—for men and women—after any serious illness.

✚ CONVENTIONAL MEDICINE

Excessive hair growth can be treated with electrolysis or waxing, but electrolysis can be expensive and waxing needs to be repeated every few months. Hair loss after pregnancy or due to *Alopecia areata* tends to regrow, although your physician may order blood tests to make sure that your thyroid gland is working normally. Male-pattern baldness can be treated, but the new hair is downy and falls out if treatment is stopped. Dandruff can be controlled with shampoo or lotion. In severe cases consult your physician.

DOSAGE: ADULTS AND CHILDREN For male-pattern baldness, apply a solution containing minoxidil twice a day. For dandruff, use a mild shampoo with tea tree oil once or twice a week. Products containing Ketoconazole are also effective. If using bleach, do a test patch first and follow directions; consult label for details.

✿ HOMEOPATHIC REMEDIES

 Graphites 6c
For crusts on scalp. Also eczema behind ears, which may be moist. Oozes sticky fluid.

 Oleander 6c
For large, white flakes falling from hair. Scalp dry or itchy. Psoriasis or cradle cap (in babies). Generally worse for eating oranges.

DOSAGE I tablet twice daily. Maximum 2 weeks.

NUTRITION

Anemia is one of the most frequent causes of hair loss, so eat plenty of iron-rich foods, like liver (not if you are pregnant), all other organ meat, whole grain cereals, dark green leafy vegetables, eggs, dates, and raisins. Vitamin C improves the absorption of iron, so eat fruit or vegetables at the same time. Vitamin E is also important for healthy hair growth, so eat avocados, nuts, seeds, and olive oil on a regular basis. Reduce your intake of animal fat and sugar, as these can aggravate the production of sebum.

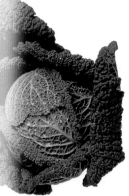

ABOVE Cabbage contains iron, which is needed to prevent anemia.

 ## HERBAL REMEDIES

Herbs have a beneficial effect on a wide range of hair problems.

USE AND DOSAGE For dandruff, add 1–2 cups of rosemary or stinging-nettle infusion to the final rinse when shampooing. Avoid if you are pregnant.

Hair loss will sometimes respond to arnica, or southernwood (gently massage an infused oil into the scalp).

For dry hair, take marshmallow and burdock as a tea (1tsp of each per cup). Avoid if you are pregnant. For itchiness, use a final rinse of catmint or chamomile infusion.

AROMATHERAPY

- Rosemary *(Rosmarinus officinalis)*
- Roman chamomile *(Chamaemelum nobile)*
- Lemon *(Citrus limon)*
- Grapefruit *(Citrus x paradisi)*
- Cedarwood *(Cedrus atlantica)*

Rosemary is usually used for dark hair and chamomile for fair. Lemon, grapefruit, and cedarwood stimulate the circulation and balance the body's secretions, thereby reducing dandruff. Avoid using rosemary if you are pregnant.

APPLICATION Add 2 drops of essential oil to the rinse water, then massage into the scalp. Wrap your hair in plastic wrap, then place a warm towel around it and leave for 2–3 hours. Then use a mild shampoo (not medicated), to avoid damaging the sebum balance.

Caution

Avoid rosemary oil if you have high blood pressure; if you have sensitive skin, keep lemon and grapefruit doses low as they may be irritant.

BELOW Add grapefruit oil to the final rinsing water when washing your hair to reduce dandruff.

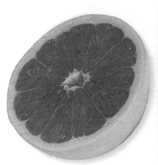

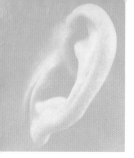

Earache

Throbbing pain and fever, often during or after a cold; may be worse in an airplane; child may scream and pull at one ear—likely causes: middle-ear infection or congestion; pain after syringing or swimming—likely cause: external ear infection.

arache is a common problem, especially in young children, and is generally caused by an infection. The Eustachian tube, which links the back of the nose and throat to the middle ear, can allow bacteria access to this sensitive region. The lining of the ear canal is very thin and easily damaged if you scratch or clean it overenthusiastically; an infected ear canal will be sore and often produces a discharge. Earache in children should always be regarded as serious and seen by your physician, although it is not necessary to resort to antibiotics every time. Home remedies often avoid the need for stronger medication.

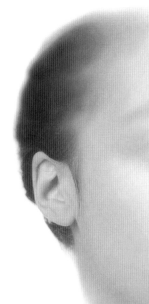

🔵 Call the physician
If earache persists in young children; if you have severe earache.

 CONVENTIONAL MEDICINE

To prevent damage to the ear canal, avoid cleaning the ears with cotton swabs or scratching them too vigorously. A pain reliever will usually ease earache, but if the pain persists or if you have noticed any discharge from the ear, consult your physician. In the meantime, keep the ear dry by putting cotton in it while showering.

DOSAGE: ADULTS 1–2 tablets of pain relievers at onset of pain, repeated every 4 hours; consult label for details.

DOSAGE: CHILDREN Give regular doses of children's pain reliever; consult label, or follow medical advice.

 HERBAL REMEDIES

It is very important to avoid putting anything in the ear if there is the slightest risk that the eardrum has been perforated.

USE AND DOSAGE Warmed herbal oils (infused mullein or St. John's wort, for instance) can be helpful as ear drops.

Alternatively, you can infuse a chamomile teabag for a few minutes, then place it over the ear while it is still warm.

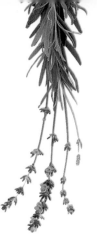

HOMEOPATHIC REMEDIES

For recurrent earache, consult a qualified homeopath; if worsening, consult a physician.

⚬ Pulsatilla 6c

For heavy, pressing pain outward from eardrum. Worse for applied heat. Thick, bland, smelly discharge. Child is miserable, clingy, and wants cuddles.

⚬ Chamomilla 6c

For severe, sharp pains in the ear driving person frantic. Child is irritable, angry, better for moving.

⚬ Belladonna 6c

For sudden onset. Throbbing earache worse for heat. Hypersensitive hearing. Face very hot and red. Skin dry, may be delirious.

⚬ Aconite 6c

For initial stages of earache. Pains may be worse in left ear.

DOSAGE 1 tablet every 4 hours for 2–3 days or until better.

ABOVE Lavender is a highly soothing oil and will help dull the pain of earache.

AROMATHERAPY

⚬ Lavender (Lavandula angustifolia)
⚬ Roman chamomile (Chamaemelum nobile)

Chamomile is beneficial for a dull ache and lavender for sharp pain.

APPLICATION Put a drop of lavender on some cotton, then make a plug to place in the ear. Use chamomile in a warm compress on the side of the face.

Caution

Do not pour essential oil directly into the ear. If pus appears from the ear or you develop a fever, seek medical help. Always read pain-reliever packs carefully, and do not exceed the stated dose.

NUTRITION

Children with recurrent earache may respond to a diet free of dairy products for a short period, as this seems to reduce the amount of mucus. But if your child is on such a diet, seek professional advice to ensure there are no nutritional deficiencies.

Pineapple juice should be drunk for its healing enzymes, and citrus juices for their vitamin C. Most children will want little food apart from light snacks, as swallowing often worsens the pain. For adults, decongestant spices, such as cinnamon, ginger, chili, and mustard, will help. Avoid cinnamon and chili if you are pregnant and ginger if you have gallstones.

CINNAMON

MUSTARD

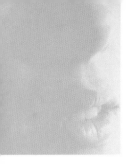

Bad breath: halitosis

*An unpleasant smell on the breath; usually due to poor
dental hygiene, but may also be caused by sinus infection
or congestion, digestive disorders, constipation, the
underproduction of saliva,, smoking, and drinking alcohol.*

Medically, bad breath is not usually very significant. Sometimes,
however, it can be an indication of a more serious illness, such as
liver failure, kidney disease, or diabetes. Halitosis can occur as the
result of bad dental hygiene—a build-up of plaque, infected gums, a
tooth abscess, a rotting filling, or lazy brushing. People often become
obsessive about their breath, but dentists now have electronic devices
that measure the odors in exhaled breath. More people lose their teeth
through gum disease than tooth decay *(see Gingivitis on p.150)*, so prac-
ticing good dental hygiene is important for more than just fresh breath.

✚ CONVENTIONAL MEDICINE

Looking after teeth and gums by regular brushing,
flossing, and dental check-ups will help ensure that
they are not responsible for unpleasant smells in
the mouth. Sensible eating habits will often avoid
the problem, but it is important to seek medical
advice if there is no obvious cause.

HERBAL REMEDIES

Identifying the cause of bad breath is important.
USE AND DOSAGE If hyperacidity is to blame,
then meadowsweet tea can help. Do not
use if you are sensitive to aspirin. If sluggish
digestion is at fault, then use agrimony or fenugreek seeds (1tsp of herb to a cup of boiling water).
Where bad breath is associated with sinus congestion, use a tea-tree oil inhalant.
A traditional remedy is to chew a few lovage or
fennel seeds. Avoid fennel if you are pregnant and
lovage if you have a heart or kidney problem.
An effective herbal mouth spray can be made
by adding 1tsp each of tea-tree and rosemary oils
to ½ cup of water and then pouring the mixture
into a spray bottle. Avoid if you are pregnant.

ABOVE Don't just mask
bad breath; improve oral
hygiene to eliminate it.

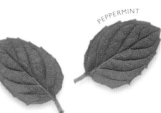

PEPPERMINT

AROMATHERAPY

- Tea tree *(Melaleuca alternifolia)*
- Peppermint *(Mentha x piperita)*
- Thyme *(Thymus vulgaris)*
- Lemon *(Citrus limon)*
- Niaouli *(Melaleuca viridiflora)*

These oils kill off any unnecessary bacteria or viral infection in the mouth or throat that might be responsible for bad breath. Avoid peppermint if you have a gallbladder or liver problem.

APPLICATION Use in a mouthwash or gargle.

HOMEOPATHIC REMEDIES

Make sure that there is no serious cause for this particular complaint.

- Pulsatilla 6c

For halitosis in the morning. Dry mouth with greasy taste. Not thirsty. Food may taste bitter.

- Kali bichromicum 6c

For offensive breath, sensation of a hair on the tongue. Thick saliva, ropy, yellow phlegm.

DOSAGE I tablet twice daily. Maximum 2 weeks.

NUTRITION

Constipation is thought to be a common cause of bad breath and is easily remedied *(see p.96)*. Sinus infections, congestion, and chronic chest diseases can also be responsible *(see Congestion on p.42, Sinusitis on p.50)*. Some people find the smell of garlic, onions, curries, and other highly spiced food unpleasant, although all these foods are healthy—so avoid them if you feel you must. Daily helpings of natural live yogurt, plenty of water, and adequate amounts of fiber-containing foods all improve the digestive function and will help bad breath. Eat broccoli, spinach, and citrus fruits for their beta-carotene and vitamin C. Ginger, mustard, and cinnamon are good for the sinuses; cut down on dairy products to reduce mucus. Avoid ginger if you have gallstones. Chewing caraway seeds, mint leaves, or parsley may help. Avoid cinnamon and parsley if you are pregnant and parsley if you have a heart or kidney condition.

> **Caution**
> *Do not give mouthwashes containing essential oils to children.*

BELOW If bad breath is caused by poor digestion, boost the immune system by increasing your intake of high-fiber foods.

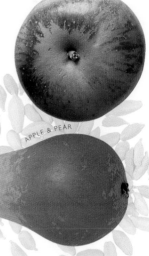

APPLE & PEAR

Canker sores

Painful white craters, often with bright red borders, which may occur singly or in clusters and often recur; may appear on the tongue, the roof of the mouth, the groove between the gums and cheek, or elsewhere on the cheek.

anker sores, or mouth ulcers, are painful, irritating sore patches found inside the mouth, usually on the inside of the lips (especially the lower one) and cheeks, but also on the gums and roof of the mouth. The medical term for canker sores is apthous ulcers, and though they are frequently caused by injury—from biting the cheek or lip, badly fitting dentures, or the jagged edge of a damaged tooth—in some cases, there is no clear cause. Rarely, mouth ulcers are associated with an underlying disorder affecting the whole digestive tract.

🌐 Call the dentist

If you have an ulcer that recurs regularly in the same place, as it is quite likely to be caused by a dental problem; if an ulcer fails to heal after 3 weeks.

 CONVENTIONAL MEDICINE

Most ulcers improve with no treatment after a few days, but may last for 2 weeks. Treatments include topical anesthetic ointments to relieve the pain, protective gels, and a prescription steroid paste to speed healing. Avoid hot, spicy, or acidic foods.

DOSAGE: ADULTS AND CHILDREN Apply a local anesthetic ointment, combined with the steroid paste, if necessary, to the ulcer at regular intervals; consult labels for details. Saltwater mouthwashes used three or four times a day may be helpful.

 AROMATHERAPY

Myrrh *(Commiphora molmol)*
Myrrh helps to kill the pain and the infection, and stop it from spreading. If you cannot get hold of myrrh essential oil, then myrrh tincture can be used instead of the myrrh and vodka solution.

APPLICATION Put 2 drops of myrrh in 1 tsp of vodka, then dab directly onto the mouth ulcer.

 HERBAL REMEDIES

Suitable herbs for mouthwashes include marigold, raspberry leaves, cloves, or chamomile.

USE AND DOSAGE Myrrh and goldenseal can be very

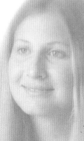
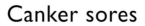

effective mouthwashes: buy the tinctures from a pharmacy or health-food store and add 10–20 drops of either to a glass of warm water. Avoid goldenseal if you are pregnant.

Strengthen the immune system with regular garlic capsules to help recurrent ulcer problems.

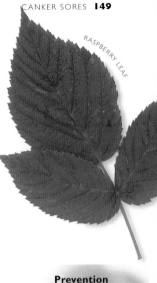

RASPBERRY LEAF

NUTRITION

As this condition is so often related to stress, it is important to eat a diet that is extra-rich in all the B vitamins, so make sure that you eat plenty of meat, poultry, wheat germ, brewer's yeast, leafy green vegetables, whole grain cereals, and whole wheat bread. Avoid foods that may be damaging to the delicate mucous membranes of the mouth, including very salty food, such as chips, salted nuts, vinegar, pickles, chilis, and very hot curries. If you have mouth ulcers, all these foods will make them much more painful. Chilis should be avoided if you are pregnant.

An effective natural remedy is to cut a clove of garlic in half, squeeze it until the oils appear, then dab it on the canker sore two or three times a day. Although this treatment stings and smells, the sore will normally disappear within 24 hours.

Prevention

Regular sufferers of mouth ulcers should take a daily dose of 5,000 IU of vitamin A, 200mg of vitamin E, and 10mg of vitamin B_2. It is also helpful to suck a combined vitamin C and zinc lozenge every day.

HOMEOPATHIC REMEDIES

Check with your physician that there is no anemia. Consult a homeopath to treat the tendency toward ulcers.

Borax 6c

For painful, white ulcers that bleed easily on contact, or when eating. Mouth hot and tender. Bitter taste in mouth.

Nitric acid 6c

For blisters and ulcers in mouth that bleed easily. Ulcers on tongue and soft palate. Tongue clean, red.

Natrum muriaticum 6c

For recurrent mouth ulcers, cold sores, and colds. Person may be introverted and easily hurt.

DOSAGE 1 tablet twice daily until improved. Maximum 5 days.

BELOW Spicy or salty food can irritate canker sores, so try to avoid it.

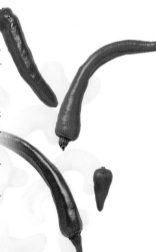

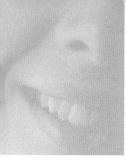

Gingivitis

Characterized by sore gums, which may be red and bleed easily when you clean your teeth; associated with tartar and plaque around the margin of the gum; needs treating to prevent eventual loss of teeth.

Far more teeth are lost through gum disease than through tooth decay, and gingivitis—a condition in which the gums bleed very easily, and dental plaque and tartar accumulate around the gum margin—is by far the most common form of gum disease. If gingivitis is left untreated, pockets of infected pus can develop at the base of teeth, followed eventually by abscesses and loose teeth, which may in time fall out. Good oral hygiene is essential to the prevention of this painful condition, but home remedies can make an extremely effective cure once infection occurs.

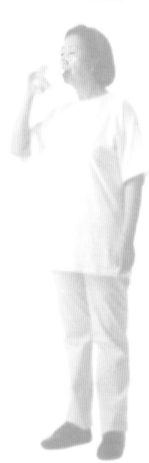

CONVENTIONAL MEDICINE

Antiseptic mouthwashes and pain-relievers may help in the first instance. Seek the advice of a dentist or hygienist if the symptoms persist.

DOSAGE: ADULTS 1–2 tablets of pain-relievers at onset of pain, repeated every 4 hours; consult label. Use a recommended mouthwash twice a day.

DOSAGE: CHILDREN Give regular doses of children's pain-reliever; consult label, or follow medical advice. Use a recommended mouthwash twice a day.

AROMATHERAPY

- Myrrh *(Commiphora molmol)*
- Tea tree *(Melaleuca alternifolia)*
- Thyme *(Thymus vulgaris)*

These oils are all healing and help to stop infection; thyme is antiseptic and myrrh is antimicrobial; tea tree helps build up the body's immune system.

APPLICATION Use in a mouthwash, putting a few drops of essential oil into a cup of warm water. Alternatively, massage myrrh tincture into the gums to improve the circulation (make sure your hands are very clean before you do this to avoid the spread of infection).

NUTRITION

It is the fibrous, as well as the nutritional, content of your food that is important in treating gingivitis. The massaging effect of biting on apples, pears, celery, and raw carrots stimulates the blood flow to the margins of the gums and prevents the development of plaque, which is a haven for bacteria. Unfortunately, when this condition develops, the gums bleed easily, making the consumption of raw foods quite painful, and so a vicious circle starts.

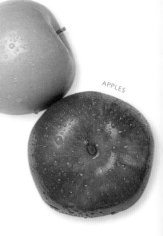
APPLES

Eat plentiful daily amounts of citrus fruits and all other fresh produce for their vitamin C. Eat as little sugar as possible and try to clean your teeth immediately after eating any high-sugar foods. If this is not possible, then chewing sugar-free gum for 15 minutes will help. And 1tsp of salt added to a glass of hot water makes a cheap, effective mouthwash.

 HOMEOPATHIC REMEDIES

Mercurius solubilis 6c
For inflamed, bleeding gums. Produces lots of saliva. Breath is offensive and teeth may be loose. Metallic taste in mouth. Mouth moist but person is thirsty.

Phosphorus 6c
For gums that bleed easily and ulcerate. Bleeding after tooth extraction.

Nitric acid 6c
For teeth that become loose; spongy, bleeding gums. Tongue clean, red. May have ulcers on palate.
DOSAGE 1 tablet three times daily.
Maximum 1 week.

Caution
Some mouthwashes may cause brown stains on the teeth, which will improve when the mouthwash is stopped.

BELOW Supplement your oral-hygiene routine with an herbal mouthwash.

 HERBAL REMEDIES

Herbal mouthwashes can help to tone and improve gum tissues.
USE AND DOSAGE Use a cooled, well-strained infusion or decoction containing herbs like lady's mantle, marigold, marjoram, or tormentil (2tsp per cup). Do not give marjoram to babies or small children.

Take goldenseal capsules to boost the immune system. Avoid if you are pregnant.

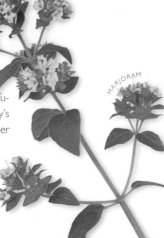
MARJORAM

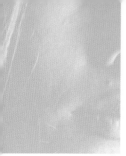

Toothache

Pain around a tooth; short bursts of pain, with inflammation of tooth pulp—likely cause: caries; long periods of pain, or sudden, severe pain—likely cause: inflamed pulp; intense, throbbing pain with sensitive gum—likely cause: abscess.

Toothache is usually the result of poor dental hygiene. Scrupulous attention to oral hygiene—proper flossing, careful brushing, and a reduced consumption of canned soft drinks and sugar in general—represents the first step. Next come regular visits to your dentist. But many of the problems associated with toothache can be avoided by healthy eating. Dental caries (tooth decay), an abscess, or gingivitis (see p.150) may be the cause of the pain. See your dentist! Weeks of painkillers will keep you going until the tooth pulp dies off and the pain stops, but then you will almost certainly lose the tooth.

Caution
Always read pain-reliever labels carefully, and do not exceed the stated dose.

 CONVENTIONAL MEDICINE

Take a pain-reliever as necessary to ease the toothache, and contact your dentist.
DOSAGE: ADULTS 1–2 tablets of pain-relievers at onset, repeated every 4 hours; consult label.
DOSAGE: CHILDREN Give regular doses of liquid pain-reliever; consult label, or follow medical advice.

 HOMEOPATHIC REMEDIES

This condition requires dental assessment by a qualified practitioner.

Chamomilla 30c
Teething remedy for children. Person is intensely irritable, has intolerable pains, and cries angrily. Child has to be carried constantly. Better for warm food.

Plantago 30c
For teeth that are sore to touch, swelling in cheeks. Produces a lot of saliva. Worse for cold air and contact. Better for eating.

Magnesium carbonicum 30c
For toothache in pregnancy. Teeth very sensitive to touch. Worse at night. Pain from cutting wisdom teeth.
DOSAGE 1 tablet hourly for six doses, as needed.

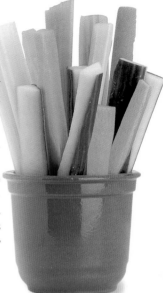

 ### NUTRITION

Good oral hygiene is the key to avoiding dental problems, although healthy eating can help. Eat plentiful daily amounts of citrus fruits and all other fresh produce, as vitamin C is the most important single nutrient in combating gum disease; crisp foods like apples, raw carrots, and celery, which massage the gums when you chew; olive oil, sunflower-seed oil, and sprouted seeds for their vitamin A; carrots, dark green leafy vegetables, and liver (in limited quantities or not at all if you are pregnant) for their vitamin A. Reduce your intake of sugar, which is your gums' worst enemy—eat as little as possible and try to clean your teeth immediately after you eat any high-sugar foods.

 ### HERBAL REMEDIES

For abscesses and similar infections, strong antibiotic herbs—especially Chinese figwort (Xuan Shen), forsythia berries—can sometimes solve the problem completely.

USE AND DOSAGE These antibiotic herbs are best taken in tinctures (1 tsp three times daily).

ABOVE Crunchy vegetables such as celery can help to improve the condition of your gums.

AROMATHERAPY

❧ Clove *(Syzygium aromaticum)*
❧ Roman chamomile *(Chamaemelum nobile)*

These oils represent only first-aid help until you can see your dentist. Clove has an anesthetic effect and is also a strong antiseptic. Chamomile is soothing and helps to kill the pain.

APPLICATION Dip a piece of cotton into some clove oil, roll it into a ball and apply it to the painful part of the tooth. You can also rub clove oil around the gum, or even hold a clove in the mouth. If you have mild toothache, then a warm chamomile compress on the facial area is very soothing.

Prevention
Good oral hygiene, low consumption of sugars and high-sugar foods, and healthy eating are all you need to prevent tooth problems leading to toothache.

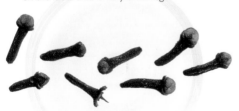

LEFT Cloves can provide a drug-free alternative treatment for toothache.

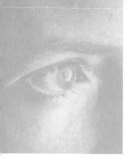

Conjunctivitis

Typical symptoms are eyes that have a red or puffy appearance, and a gritty feeling; a watery or sticky discharge; eyes that are often itchy; symptoms may affect either one or both eyes.

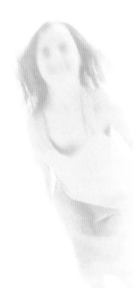

onjunctivitis, commonly called pinkeye, is an acute inflammation of the conjunctiva—the mucous membrane that covers the whites of the eyes and the inner surface of the eyelids. The condition is caused by an infection or allergy, although a foreign body in the eye can result in the appearance of similar symptoms. Conjunctivitis can be serious and is highly contagious, particularly in close-knit communities.

 CONVENTIONAL MEDICINE

For minor infections, bathe the eyes with water that has been boiled and then cooled. If this does not help, then antibiotic drops or ointment may be helpful. For allergic conjunctivitis, antihistamine eyedrops can ease the symptoms.

DOSAGE: ADULTS AND CHILDREN Pull down the lower lid and insert antibiotics or ointment; consult labels for details, or follow medical advice. Continue the treatment for 48 hours after the symptoms have resolved themselves.

 HOMEOPATHIC REMEDIES

If the following remedies produce no improvement, seek medical help.

❧ Apis 6c

For swollen, red, puffy eyelids. White of eye red, hot tears, intolerance of light.

❧ Argentum nitricum 6c

For yellow or white discharge, white of eye red. Babies with sticky eye.

❧ Pulsatilla 6c

For white or yellow discharge. Lids inflamed. Itching and burning. Person may be weepy and feel sorry for themselves.

❧ Euphrasia 6c

For white of eye that is red, constantly watering. Tears burn, lids swollen.

DOSAGE I tablet every 4 hours. Maximum 2 days. Euphrasia tincture can be diluted (2 drops in an eggcup of cooled boiled water) to make a solution with which to bathe the eye.

HERBAL REMEDIES

Herbal eyebaths are soothing and easy to make. Suitable herbs are marigold flowers, eyebright, chamomile flowers, rose petals, raspberry leaves, elderflowers, and fumitory.

USE AND DOSAGE Add I tsp of herb to a cup of boiling water; simmer gently for 5 minutes before straining well. Allow to cool and use in an eyebath.

Take echinacea (5 x 200mg capsules every day) to combat any infection. Avoid if you are pregnant or breastfeeding, or have a disorder of the immune system.

AROMATHERAPY

No essential oils can be used in the vicinity of the eyes.

NUTRITION

Foods that are rich in beta-carotene, which the body converts to vitamin A, are important for all eye conditions—so eat orange and red fruits, all dark green leafy vegetables, carrots, and liver (in limited quantities or not at all if you are pregnant). Thin slices of cucumber or used, cold teabags placed over the closed eyes for 6 minutes will help to relieve the inflammation caused by conjunctivitis.

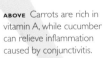

ABOVE Carrots are rich in vitamin A, while cucumber can relieve inflammation caused by conjunctivitis.

Prevention

Avoid touching the eyes as much as possible; wash hands often; don't share towels or eye makeup. Protect your eyes by wearing suitable goggles for do-it-yourself projects.

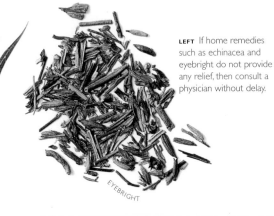

ECHINACEA

EYEBRIGHT

LEFT If home remedies such as echinacea and eyebright do not provide any relief, then consult a physician without delay.

Styes

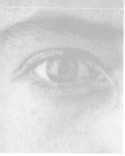

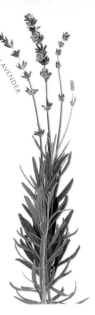

Starts with a painful lump near an eyelash; the pain may become severe and throbbing and the stye may discharge pus.

LAVENDER

A stye is an abscess in the tiny gland that is located at the bottom of each eyelash. It comes to a head or "point" on the outside of the lid and can cause extreme inflammation of the eyelids. Infection may spread to the eye itself, so styes are not to be treated lightly. They tend to be more common in those who have low resistance and those in poor general health.

CONVENTIONAL MEDICINE

A stye will often get better with no treatment except pain-relievers or warm compresses. If it does not, then a course of antibiotics may be necessary.

DOSAGE: ADULTS 1–2 tablets of pain-relievers at onset, repeated every 4 hours.

DOSAGE: CHILDREN Give regular doses of children's pain-reliever; consult label or follow medical advice.

HERBAL REMEDIES

Marigold or eyebright decoctions can be used to bathe the affected area; a little marigold cream may also help.

USE AND DOSAGE Simmer the decoction for 5 minutes to ensure a sterile mixture for bathing the eye.

If styes are recurrent and linked to overwork, take Siberian ginseng in the buildup to any especially stressful period (avoid if you are pregnant).

HOMEOPATHIC REMEDIES

 Staphysagria 6c

For recurrent styes, and styes that leave a hard, inflamed area in the skin.

DOSAGE 1 tablet every 4 hours until stye is improved. Maximum 4 days.

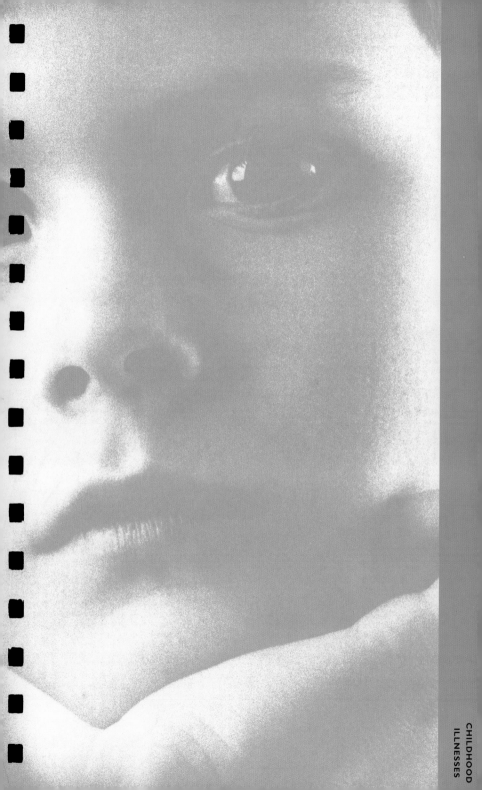

Childhood
Illnesses

Children are naturally resilient, but all of them at one time or another fall prey to illnesses like tonsillitis, measles, or whooping cough, and there is nothing more miserable than seeing a child in discomfort and feeling that there is little you can do to help. However, although conventional medicine (particularly vaccination) has an important role to play, there is much else that you can do at home to help alleviate these conditions. And even before illness takes hold, you can raise a child's resistance to infection and boost natural immunity.

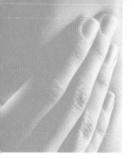

Tonsillitis

A sore throat, accompanied by difficulty in swallowing; swollen glands in the neck; a coated tongue; fever; the tonsils themselves may be red and inflamed, and covered in yellow spots of pus.

Tonsillitis is an acute infection of the tonsils, usually caused by a virus, although it may be bacterial. When the tonsils become infected they look red and angry, but they are simply doing their job—trapping invading organisms before you inhale them. Tonsillitis occurs mostly in children, especially when first exposed to a range of bugs on starting school. Sometimes the problem becomes chronic, and it may also affect adults. Severe infections may need treatment with antibiotics (which are only effective against bacterial infections), but home remedies are a powerful aid to reducing pain and speedier healing.

BELOW Children might need antibiotics to ward off severe tonsillitis.

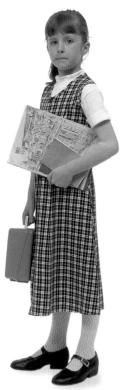

 CONVENTIONAL MEDICINE

Most infections will improve without any treatment, but physicians prescribe antibiotics for bacterial infections if symptoms have been present for several days. Painkillers can relieve the sore throat and fever (but do not give aspirin), and can be dissolved to produce an anesthetic gargle. Lozenges and hot drinks can be soothing. Recurrent infections may be prevented by surgery to remove the tonsils.

DOSAGE: ADULTS Antibiotic tablets up to four times a day; follow medical advice; complete the course.

DOSAGE: CHILDREN Give antibiotics as prescribed. Dose depends on age and weight of child; follow medical advice; complete the course.

NUTRITION

During a bout of tonsillitis swallowing can be very painful, so give blended vegetable soups made with carrots, sweet potatoes, and broccoli for their beta-carotene; shredded cabbage and tomatoes for their vitamin C; and leeks, onions, and garlic for their antiseptic qualities. Crush 2 peeled cloves of garlic into a jar of runny honey; give a teaspoonful every two hours. (Do not give honey to children under two.)

Drink plenty of hot water, honey, and lemon, together with unsweetened fruit juices. Home-made ice pops of pure frozen pineapple juice are easy to suck, and the bromelain in the pineapple helps reduce both the swollen glands and tonsils.

HERBAL REMEDIES

Mild cases of tonsillitis will generally respond well to gargling with sage and echinacea tinctures (1tsp of each) diluted in a glass of warmed pineapple juice (but do not use if your child has a specific disorder of the immune system).

Raspberry-leaf tea is another suitable gargle that can be used for children.

USE AND DOSAGE Support the immune system with echinacea capsules (up to 600mg four times a day), but, again, not if you child has a specific disorder of the immune system.

HOMEOPATHIC REMEDIES

Recurrent problems are best treated by a homeopath.

Phytolacca 30c

For dark red or purple tonsils with gray or white pus. Pain goes to ear on swallowing. Worse on right side, worse for warm drinks. Better for cold drinks.

Lachesis 30c

For purple tonsils. Wakes with sore throat or worse after sleep. Worse on left side, for swallowing liquids and saliva. May start on left side and move to right.

DOSAGE 1 tablet every 2 hours for three doses, then every 4 hours. Maximum 2 days.

AROMATHERAPY

Thyme (Thymus vulgaris)

Lavender (Lavandula angustifolia)

Tea tree (Melaleuca alternifolia)

Tea tree and thyme both fight the infection; lavender and thyme have a slightly anesthetic effect.

APPLICATION Use in steam inhalations or in a warm compress on the throat area. If other symptoms occur, such as earache, headache, or abdominal pain, then look under the appropriate ailment.

 Call the physician
If you you are unable to swallow saliva; if a non-teething child drools.

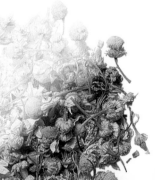
BELOW Try chamomile teas as a healing drink, or for gargling.

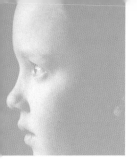

Measles

*Characterized by a fever; runny nose; red, watery eyes; cough;
and swollen glands. After 3–4 days an itchy rash develops,
starting at the head and spreading downward, fading
after 3 days.*

**This highly contagious viral infection causes a rash and attacks the
respiratory system. The concerted effort to vaccinate all school
children now makes it a much rarer complaint than it used to be, but it
is still a very serious illness and should not be taken lightly. Home
remedies are not a substitute for your physician's advice, but they can
make a child much more comfortable. Children with measles must be
isolated; the infectious period lasts from the first symptoms—congestion, conjunctivitis, high fever, and complete misery—until 5 days after
the first appearance of the rash. It can take up to 3 weeks to develop
symptoms after being in contact with someone who has measles.**

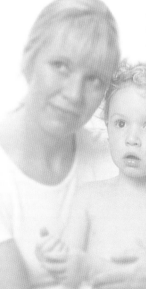

 CONVENTIONAL MEDICINE

Treat the fever with pain relievers and use calamine
lotion to soothe itchy skin.

DOSAGE: ADULTS 1–2 tablets of pain relievers at
onset of fever, repeated every 4 hours; consult label
for details. Apply calamine lotion/cream directly to
the skin as required.

DOSAGE: CHILDREN Give regular doses of children's
pain reliever (do not use aspirin); consult label for
details, or follow medical advice. Apply calamine
lotion/cream directly to the skin as required.

 HERBAL REMEDIES

Herbs can ease symptoms and combat the infection, to support orthodox treatments.

USE AND DOSAGE To soothe coughs and throats,
make an infusion of equal parts of hyssop, marshmallow, catmint, and English plantain (½–1 tsp of the
mix per cup, depending on child's age) and sweeten
with a little honey (not for children under two).

Use well-strained, cooled infusions of eyebright
or self-heal to bathe sore eyes, or to soak a cloth
for use as a compress.

Use lemon-balm tea to help reduce fevers.

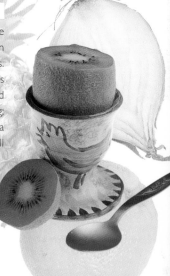

NUTRITION

Few children with measles will feel like eating in the early stages, but as soon as they do, foods rich in vitamins A and C should be given as light meals. Puréed carrot with a poached egg; sweet potatoes cut into chips and roasted; dried apricots puréed with yogurt and stirred into gelatin before setting; kiwi fruit with their tops sliced off and eaten like a boiled egg…these foods are easy to eat and will boost the immune system and protect the eyes.

Fruit juices—especially pineapple and orange—should be given in large amounts, diluted 50:50 with water. And leeks, garlic, and onions are all protective against the secondary chest infection that often accompanies measles.

HOMEOPATHIC REMEDIES

If the condition worsens, consult a physician.

Morbillinum 30c

After contact with measles, this remedy may help to prevent the disease. Take every 8 hours, 3 doses only.

Bryonia 6c

For dryness, hotness. Cough with headache. Worse for any motion. May be used before rash appears.

Pulsatilla 6c

For miserable, clingy child, who wants to be cuddled. Bland, creamy discharge from eyes. Not thirsty. Temperature not very high.

DOSAGE I tablet every 4 hours until improved. Maximum 5 days.

AROMATHERAPY

Tea tree (Melaleuca alternifolia)
Roman chamomile (Chamaemelum nobile)
Lavender (Lavandula angustifolia)

These essential oils help to fight infection and are also soothing.

APPLICATION Vaporize the sickroom to stop the virus from spreading through the air. Use the oils with a little warm water to sponge down the patient, or to spray into the air. Also use them as inhalations, especially if there is a sore throat.

ABOVE Tempt convalescing children with foods that are easy—and fun—to eat.

Caution

Watch out for convulsions caused by very high fevers and for the possibility of meningitis, eye problems, and secondary infections. Read pain reliever labels carefully, and do not exceed the stated dose. Take Morbillinum for three doses only.

German measles: rubella

Mild fever; sore throat; and swollen glands, particularly behind the ears; the rash lasts 2–3 days, usually starting on the face and spreading downward; individual spots may join together to produce a more generally flushed skin.

he only significant thing about this mild, infectious disease is the risk it carries in pregnancy. Today most children are vaccinated against rubella (the medical term), but any child who does catch German measles must be kept away from all pregnant women, because of the risk to the unborn fetus—including deafness, blindness, heart and lung defects, and even death. Many women in the earliest stages of pregnancy may be unaware they are pregnant. Children with the illness must be kept at home during the infectious period, which lasts from the start of symptoms until at least 1 week after the rash appears.

 Call the physician
If German measles is suspected; if you are pregnant, have been in contact with rubella and are not sure of your immune status.

 CONVENTIONAL MEDICINE

If you have this common viral infection, you should rest if you feel unwell and avoid contact with other people, particularly school-age children and pregnant women. Although most women have had rubella or been immunized, if you are pregnant and worried that you have the illness, or have been in contact with someone with rubella, you should contact your physician.

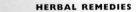 **HERBAL REMEDIES**

Plenty of fluids are needed and herbal teas are ideal: they can be sweetened or flavored with honey (not for children under two) or lemon. Many soothing, cooling herbs are suitable, including hyssop.

USE AND DOSAGE Elderflowers, marigold, and chamomile make a good combination; use ½–2tsp per cup of water (depending on age).

Echinacea capsules (100–600mg daily) will help combat the infection of German measles (but do not use if you child has a specific disorder of the immune system).

Agrimony or cleavers tea helps to ease sore throats and swollen glands.

AROMATHERAPY

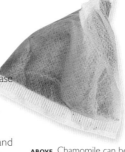

- Lavender *(Lavandula angustifolia)*
- Roman chamomile *(Chamaemelum nobile)*
- Tea tree *(Melaleuca alternifolia)*

Chamomile and lavender can be used to help ease any irritation from the rash. Tea tree, when burned or vaporized, helps to prevent the virus from spreading.

APPLICATION Use a few drops of chamomile and lavender in the bath; add them under running water. They can also be used (as can tea tree) in warm water to sponge children down, if they are getting clammy and distressed. Burn or vaporize the tea tree oil; alternatively use it in a water spray in the sickroom.

ABOVE Chamomile can be used to ease an irritating rash or it may be added to bath water.

HOMEOPATHIC REMEDIES

This is usually a mild disease that doesn't require treatment. If an unimmunized woman becomes pregnant, taking Rubella 30c every 12 hours for three doses, then one dose every three weeks through the 12th week, may provide protection.

NUTRITION

Fluids are absolutely vital. Drink plenty of diluted fresh citrus juices for their immune-boosting vitamin C; pineapple juice for its soothing enzymes (pure, store-bought pineapple juice is fine); and herbal teas—chamomile, lime blossom, and elderflower are ideal.

Caution

If German measles is contracted during the first 3 months of pregnancy, the effects on the developing fetus can be catastrophic. Read pain-reliever labels carefully, and do not exceed the stated dose.

Prevention

There is no way to prevent German measles, apart from vaccination. But it is important, as always, to maintain your child's general immunity in as strong a state as possible.

ABOVE Sage tea makes a soothing remedy for rubella.

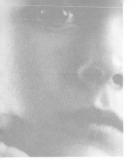

Mumps

Tiredness; mild fever; sore throat and pain on swallowing; swollen glands under the jaw; tender testicles in boys; a painful swelling in front of and below the ears after a couple of days—the temperature rises rapidly.

This highly contagious viral infection mostly affects children between the ages of 4 and 14. It starts with general malaise and fever, followed by a painful swelling of the salivary gland on one side of the face. In 70 percent of sufferers it goes on to affect the gland on the other side of the face, too. The incubation period lasts 14–21 days; sufferers are infectious (via coughs and sneezes or saliva) for 7 days before, and 9 days after, the first swelling appears. The main complication is orchitis—swelling of the testicles—which occurs in 25 percent of boys who catch the disease and can result in infertility.

 CONVENTIONAL MEDICINE

Use a simple pain reliever to reduce the fever and ease the symptoms. Eat soft food and drink plenty of liquids.

Dosage: Adults 1–2 tablets of pain relievers at onset of fever, repeated every 4 hours; consult label.

BELOW Particular care must be given to boys who contract mumps.

Dosage: Children Give regular doses of children's pain reliever (do not use aspirin); consult label for details, or follow medical advice.

 HERBAL REMEDIES

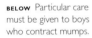

Swollen glands may be eased by a mixture of cleavers, thyme, and marigold.

Use and Dosage Mix equal amounts of the herbs and make an infusion (½–2tsp per cup, depending on the child's age); sweeten to taste with honey (not for children under two) and a tiny pinch of chili powder. Repeat every 2 hours.

Take echinacea to combat the infection (but not if you child has a specific disorder of the immune system); if the testicles are affected use chasteberry (10 drops of tincture in water three times daily).

Lemon balm infusion can be used externally in compresses applied to the face and throat.

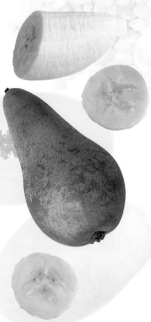

NUTRITION

Getting sufficient calories into the child is the main difficulty, and soft or blended foods and drinks are best. Give plenty of vegetable juices diluted with warm water, apple or pear juice, purées of carrot and potato, blended yogurt with honey (do not give honey to children under two), fresh non-citrus fruits like dried apricots and papayas, which are both nutritious and healing. Pineapple juice—rich in the enzyme bromelain, which is anti-inflammatory and has a high content of natural sugars—will help, too. As soon as possible, give scrambled eggs; rice or tapioca puddings; pasta; mashed potato or avocado; ice cream; minced chicken; and lots of bananas. A soluble vitamin C tablet (500mg) should be given every day. Avoid acidic fruit juices, as these increase the flow of saliva, which is very painful.

HOMEOPATHIC REMEDIES

Pulsatilla 6c
For use if the illness lingers; if there are complications of breasts swelling in girls or testicles swelling in boys (in which case, consult a physician).

Lachesis 6c
For swollen left side of face, which is sensitive to touch. Person tries to move away if someone tries to touch it. Sore throat, cannot swallow.
DOSAGE 1 tablet every 2 hours for six doses, then four times daily. Maximum 3 days.

ABOVE Blended fruit is a palatable way to tempt youngsters to eat.

AROMATHERAPY

Lavender (*Lavandula angustifolia*)
Roman chamomile (*Chamaemelum nobile*)
Tea tree (*Melaleuca alternifolia*)
Niaouli (*Melaleuca viridiflora*)
Lemon (*Citrus limon*)
Lavender and chamomile are soothing and help to kill the pain. The other oils help to combat infection.
APPLICATION Put into an oil or a lotion to smooth gently over the affected area, or use as a compress for swollen areas. Air sprays or vaporization will help stop the spread of airborne germs.

Caution
Orchitis generally affects just one testicle, with few complications, but if both testicles are severely affected there is considerable risk of sterility— seriously increased if it occurs in adults. Always read pain-reliever labels carefully, and do not exceed the stated dose.

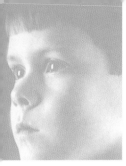

Chicken pox

Typified by low fever, vomiting, and general aches in some cases; small raised spots break out first on the trunk, then on face and limbs; clusters of itchy blisters then appear on the skin, eyes, and mouth—these gradually crust and form scabs.

This highly infectious illness is caused by the *Herpes zoster* virus and is most common in children. After contact with someone who is infected, it may be 2–3 weeks before symptoms appear. Although often just uncomfortable and irritating—the most serious side-effect is usually the scars left after picking the spots—chicken pox can be quite severe in some children. In adults, however, the infection can be extremely serious and debilitating and may lead to acute pneumonia. Those who contract chicken pox must avoid scratching, to prevent the spread of infection and the risk of scars.

 CONVENTIONAL MEDICINE

Treat the fever with pain relievers, and use calamine lotion to soothe itchy skin. More severe infections can be treated with antiviral drugs. Discuss with your physician the indications for the chicken pox vaccine.
DOSAGE: ADULTS 1–2 tablets of pain relievers at the onset of fever, repeated every 4 hours; consult label for details. Apply calamine lotion/cream directly to the skin.
DOSAGE: CHILDREN Give regular doses of children's pain reliever (do not use aspirin); consult label for details, or follow medical advice. Apply calamine lotion/cream directly to the skin as required.

 HOMEOPATHIC REMEDIES

Rhus toxicodendron 6c
For intense itching, better for warm applications. Small watery blisters. This is the first remedy to try.
Antimonium tartaricum 6c
For spots that are slow to come out. Person is drowsy, sweaty. May have a cough with a rattly chest, but does not bring up any actual mucus.
Antimonium crudum 6c
For chicken pox and upset stomach. Person is

irritable, sulky. Cries when touched, looked at, or washed. Tongue has a white coat.

DOSAGE 1 tablet every 2–4 hours until condition improves. Maximum 5 days.

HERBAL REMEDIES

Herbs can ease the fever associated with chicken pox and soothe its rash.

USE AND DOSAGE To ease fevers and irritability, use a tea made from equal parts of boneset, elderflower, and chamomile (½–2tsp per cup, depending on patient's age, three times a day).

Rashes can be soothed with a wash made by mixing borage juice (2tbsp) with standard chickweed infusion (½ cup/100ml), and distilled witch hazel (2tbsp). Apply with a cotton swab.

Taking up to 5 × 200mg echinacea capsules daily will help combat the infection (but not if your child has a specific disorder of the immune system).

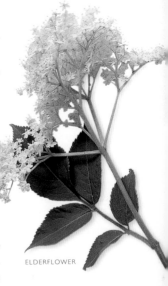

ELDERFLOWER

NUTRITION

Take plenty of fluids, especially pineapple juice—which is rich in the enzyme bromelain—diluted with water (50:50), chamomile tea, and water itself. For adults, a short fast (24–48 hours) will boost the body's white-cell count and help fight the infection.

> **Caution**
> *Always read pain-reliever labels carefully, and do not exceed the stated dose.*

AROMATHERAPY

- Lavender *(Lavandula angustifolia)*
- Roman chamomile *(Chamaemelum nobile)*
- Bergamot *(Citrus bergamia)*

Bathing in any one of these oils or rubbing in a lotion containing them will help to relieve itching. Vaporization of any of the oils will help stop the spread of the virus, so that hopefully other people will not catch it.

APPLICATION Use in lukewarm baths, vaporizers and sprays. Immerse the child in a lukewarm bath containing 1 drop of any of the above oils (but not all) every 2 hours. Regular bathing is also soothing for adults with chicken pox, who may be quite ill.

BELOW Herbal teas can soothe itching and bring down fever.

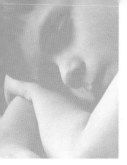

Whooping cough

Sneezing; watery red eyes; sore throat; mild fever; cough, with irregular bouts of severe coughing fits starting nearly 2 weeks later and lasting for up to 1 month; gasping for breath at the end of a coughing fit, causing the characteristic whoop.

This childhood disease is spread by coughs and sneezes and is highly infectious during the early stages. It starts with the symptoms of a normal cold, followed 2 weeks later by violent, uncontrollable bouts of coughing, which frequently end in vomiting. Because the child cannot breathe in during these spasms, they may feel as though they are suffocating, and the typical "whooping sound" is extremely distressing. In small babies, oxygen deprivation can become a real hazard. The coughing can also do permanent damage to the lungs. Home remedies can, however, speed recovery.

 CONVENTIONAL MEDICINE

If your child has been exposed to whooping cough and has not been immunized, consult your doctor and be on the lookout for symptoms, as the disease can only be treated during the first stage, before coughing fits start. Treatment is with antibiotics.

BELOW Whooping cough is a serious illness, but children can easily be immunized against it.

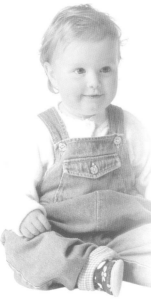

 AROMATHERAPY

- Frankincense *(Boswellia sacra)*
- Lavender *(Lavandula angustifolia)*
- Sandalwood *(Santalum album)*

Frankincense and lavender are calming and help deepen breathing. Sandalwood is antispasmodic (avoid if your child has a kidney problem).

APPLICATION Burn these oils in the sickroom, or massage the chest and back with them.

 HOMEOPATHIC REMEDIES

This is a serious condition and requires medical assessment.

- Drosera 6c

For deep spasms of coughing that start in the larynx, retching, and vomiting. Worse at night, for lying down. Better for cold drinks.

Ipecacuanha 6c
For spasmodic cough, suffocating, wheezing. Chest feels full of phlegm, but cannot cough it up. Constant feeling of nausea. Nosebleeds with cough.

Cuprum metallicum 6c
For violent, spasmodic cough with vomiting. Better for drinking water. Tight feeling in chest.
DOSAGE 1 tablet every 4 hours. Maximum 2 weeks.

HERBAL REMEDIES

Teas, such as chamomile, can help to calm the child and reduce the violent coughing spasms. They can be used to support more orthodox remedies.
USE AND DOSAGE Make a chamomile tea by pouring one-half cup of boiling water over 3 teaspoonfuls of chamomile. Cover for 5–10 minutes, and strain.

Use a chest rub of basil, hyssop, and cypress oils (2 drops of each to 1tsp of almond oil).

Wild cherry is available as a syrup.

Echinacea tablets help support the immune system (100–600mg daily in tablets, depending on age), but should be avoided if the child has a specific disorder of the immune system.

NUTRITION

It is impossible to feed normal meals to a child with severe whooping cough. Give plenty of fluids—especially if the child is vomiting. Mixtures of warm apple juice and water; pineapple and blackcurrant juice with warm water; warmed, mixed vegetable juices; warm ginger tea with honey (not for children under two or if the patient has gallstones); blended or clear soups, like vegetable or chicken broth—all these will provide nutrients. Try to avoid large amounts of milk during the first few days.

As the child begins to feel better, give small, light meals of scrambled egg; minced chicken with rice; fruit purées with cloves and cinnamon; thin porridge; puréed potato and carrot, creamed with 1–2tbsp of very low-fat yogurt. Insist on giving regular intakes of liquid, even just a couple of teaspoons at a time.

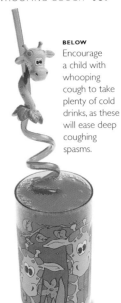
BELOW Encourage a child with whooping cough to take plenty of cold drinks, as these will ease deep coughing spasms.

Caution
Whooping cough is a serious illness, and although most children recover fully, complications can occur and medical care is essential, especially for those under the age of three.

Prevention
Avoid contact with other infected children, their siblings, or parents. The risk of contracting this disease is greatly reduced by immunization, which is safe and effective.

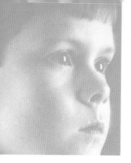

Scarlet fever

Characterized by a fever; headache; vomiting; a thick white coat to the tongue with red spots; and a red rash (which is not itchy) on various parts of the body, often accompanied by flushed red cheeks.

carlet fever is nearly always the sequel to a bout of tonsillitis in children. They will often have a sore throat, pain on swallowing, a high temperature, and inflamed tonsils, and if a rash appears 48 hours later on the neck, chest, stomach, arms, and legs, then they are almost certainly suffering from scarlet fever. A hundred years ago this was the commonest cause of death in children over the age of one year—now it is rare. It is caused by a bacterial infection and usually lasts for about a week. Scarlet fever is infectious, so make sure that you keep children away from others who are suffering from it.

 Call the physician

If you suspect someone has scarlet fever.

Caution

Scarlet fever can have serious complications, including rheumatic fever and inflammation of the kidneys, so consult a physician if in doubt or if the condition persists. Always read pain reliever labels carefully, and do not exceed the stated dose.

CONVENTIONAL MEDICINE

If you or your child show any symptoms of scarlet fever, contact your physician. If your physician confirms that you have scarlet fever, then you will need treatment with antibiotics.

DOSAGE: ADULTS 1–2 tablets of pain relievers at onset of fever, repeated every 4 hours; consult label for details.

DOSAGE: CHILDREN Consult your physician if you suspect that a child is suffering from scarlet fever; follow medical advice.

HOMEOPATHIC REMEDIES

Because of the serious complications of this disease, orthodox treatment is recommended for scarlet fever. Belladonna may, however, be used, together with orthodox medicine, to help relieve the symptoms.

Belladonna 6c

For sudden red face and high temperature; could "fry an egg" on the skin. Paleness around mouth, pupils dilated. Hallucinations.

DOSAGE 1 tablet every 2 hours for up to six doses, then every 4 hours as needed. Maximum 3 days.

NUTRITION

A sore throat and tonsillitis will make eating painful and difficult, while a high temperature means that there will be a greatly increased need for fluid replacement *(see Fever on p.16)*. Pineapple and papaya juices are of great value, as the natural enzymes that they contain are both soothing and extremely healing to the damaged and inflamed delicate membranes of the mouth and throat. Give plenty of vegetable soup made with lots of broccoli, leeks, onions, garlic, and carrots, blended and served warm in a cup. This will help boost the body's levels of the powerful antioxidant nutrients, which increase natural resistance.

PAPAYA

If antibiotics are administered, it is important to replace the natural bacteria in the digestive tract, as these will be killed off by the medication. A twice-daily drink made of a cup of live yogurt, 2tsp of honey (not for children under two), a banana, and ½ cup/120ml of milk, blended into a smooth milk-shake, should be given morning and evening.

HERBAL REMEDIES

Certain herbs can alleviate the discomfort experienced during scarlet fever.

USE AND DOSAGE Try gargles containing 10–20 drops of myrrh tincture or sage tea (2tsp per cup), to relieve a sore throat.

To help reduce fevers, drink a tea containing a mix of catmint, chamomile, elderflowers, and boneset (½–2tsp of the mix per cup, depending on the child's age).

Echinacea tablets will help combat the infection (but do not use if your child has a specific disorder of the immune system) : 100–600mg daily in tablets, depending on the child's age.

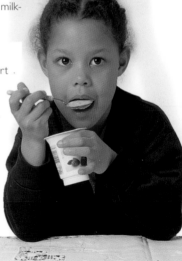

BELOW Yogurt is ideal for a child suffering from scarlet fever, since it helps to renew the beneficial bacteria that are killed off by antibiotics.

First aid

While it is important that you seek medical help for all emergencies, there are many less severe accidents and ailments that can safely be treated at home, using complementary first-aid remedies. Conventional medicine will often be the immediate standby when an accident occurs, but there are numerous herbal, homeopathic, and aromatherapeutic remedies that can help to relieve the pain of a sting or burn, calm the person who has fainted or is suffering from motion sickness, and help wounds to heal after a bruise or bite has occurred. Nutrition, in the form of kitchen medicine, has a part to play, too—honey mixed with crushed garlic, for example, makes an effective salve for cuts, while a traditional bread poultice will help to draw splinters to the surface.

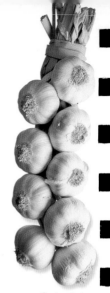

ABOVE Garlic—being antibacterial and antifungal—has a role to play in first-aid treatment.

LEFT Many minor accidents can be treated at home, but if you are in doubt about the severity of a complaint, get medical help.

Cuts

Minor cuts usually do not require medical attention, because blood clots should quickly form and seal them; but cuts should be carefully cleaned and covered with an adhesive bandage or clean dressing when the bleeding stops.

KITCHEN MEDICINE

A heaped teaspoon of salt in 2½ cups/ 600ml of warm water makes a good emergency disinfectant. A compress made from a clean cloth soaked in 2½ cups/600ml of cold water and 2tsp of vinegar is also effective. To encourage healing, crushed garlic mixed with honey and then spread thinly on a piece of clean gauze makes a great salve.

 CONVENTIONAL MEDICINE

Apply direct pressure over the cut for 10 minutes with a clean, dry cloth. If there is something stuck in the wound, such as glass, do not remove it, but apply pressure around the wound and seek medical advice. Raise the affected part of the body above chest level. If the cut is still bleeding after 10 minutes, reapply the dressing for a further 10 minutes. If the bleeding continues, apply pressure again and seek medical advice.

 HERBAL REMEDIES

After cleaning the cut with marigold infusion, apply creams or ointments containing marigold, chickweed, St. John's wort, or chamomile.

Emergency poultices can be made from crushed self-heal, woundwort, cranesbill, herb robert, agrimony, or shepherd's purse.

 AROMATHERAPY

The most relevant oils are lavender and tea tree. Clean the cut area with a bowl of warm water containing 5 drops of either oil.

BELOW Echinacea will help to prevent infection following a cut.

 HOMEOPATHIC REMEDIES

Cuts should be cleaned with water. Check that you are immunized against tetanus. Hypercal solution can be used to clean the wound, or hypercal ointment used under a clean dressing.

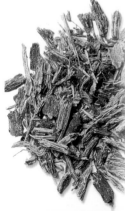

 Hypericum 30c

When injury is a puncture wound or injury to a fingertip that is rich in nerves. Pains often sharp and shooting.

DOSAGE 1 tablet every 4 hours. Maximum 3 days.

Bruises

Bruises are the visible sign of bleeding occurring beneath the skin, generally resulting either from pressure or from a blow. They usually change color over a period of several days, depending on the amount of blood below the skin.

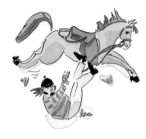

CONVENTIONAL MEDICINE

Apply an ice pack as soon as possible after the injury to reduce the swelling and bruising. Take a pain-reliever such as acetaminophen or ibuprofen.

HERBAL REMEDIES

Apply chickweed or arnica creams or lotions (but do not use arnica if the skin is broken); a cold compress soaked in sanicle, rue, or St. John's wort infusion; or a crushed cabbage leaf (held in place with an adhesive bandage if necessary).

KITCHEN MEDICINE

Pineapple juice and ice packs (*see Black Eyes opposite*) are the best kitchen medicine there is for bruises. Massaging the bruised area with a little extra-virgin olive oil will disperse the bruise, and the vitamin E that penetrates the skin is an additional aid to healing.

HOMEOPATHIC REMEDIES

Arnica 30c

The main remedy for bruises and also helpful in treating muscle aches after sport. Probably the first remedy to try. Very useful if the person does not want help and says they are okay, even when obviously they are not. Also good after surgery.

Bellis perennis 30c

For bruising that is deeper and for very sore muscles.

Ledum 30c

For very dark bruising. Area feels cold and is better for a cold compress.

DOSAGE 1 tablet every 2 hours for six doses, then three times daily. Maximum 5 days.

AROMATHERAPY

Put 4 drops of lavender and chamomile (2 drops of each) into a bowl of hot water and 2 drops of each into a bowl of cold water. Soak a facecloth in each bowl, then apply alternately to the bruised area—put the hot cloth on and when that is cool, replace with the cold one; then repeat the process.

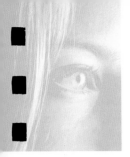

Black eyes

A black eye is the result of severe bruising of the eye socket and lids. It is internal bleeding that causes the swelling and the skin to turn black or dark blue. Sadly, most black eyes are sustained through accident or anger.

 CONVENTIONAL MEDICINE

Apply an ice pack as soon as possible after the injury to reduce the swelling and bruising. Take a pain-reliever such as acetaminophen or ibuprofen.

 HERBAL REMEDIES

Apply fresh mashed plantain leaves, or a cold compress soaked in rue infusion.

 AROMATHERAPY

Put 1 drop of chamomile into 2tsp of ice-cold water, soak a cotton-gauze pad, then apply to the affected area.

 HOMEOPATHIC REMEDIES

Several remedies are effective for the treatment of black eyes.

 Aconite 30c

Give immediately for the "shock" of the blow (can also be given for any sudden injury). One or two doses only, over 15 minutes.

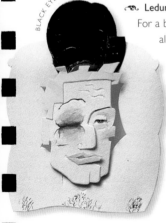

Ledum 30c

For a black eye that is generally better for cold compresses. The skin around the eye is usually swollen.

DOSAGE 1 tablet taken every 30 minutes for six doses, then repeat the dose every 2–4 hours. Maximum 12 doses.

BLACK EYE

 KITCHEN MEDICINE

The best kitchen medicine is not the old-fashioned remedy of a raw steak, but to drink copious amounts of pineapple juice— preferably before the injury (if you're a boxer); but even after the event, the enzymes in pineapple juice speed up the rate at which the blood causing the black eye dissolves, so that it will heal more quickly. A clean dish towel filled with crushed ice and placed over the area also hastens healing.

Caution

Two black eyes after a blow to the head may be the sign of a skull fracture— seek urgent medical advice.

Bites

*If the skin is punctured—whether by an animal or human
bite—wash the area well with soap and water, then see a
doctor without delay for a tetanus shot (if your immunization
isn't up to date), antibiotics, or rabies treatment, if needed.*

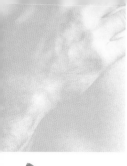
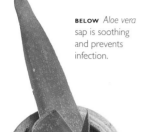

BELOW *Aloe vera*
sap is soothing
and prevents
infection.

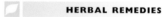

CONVENTIONAL MEDICINE

A bite from any animal (including a human bite) is
highly vulnerable to infection, as all animals have
germs in their mouths. After cleaning the wound
carefully with soap and water, dry and then cover it
with an adhesive bandage or a small sterile dressing,
then seek medical attention.

HERBAL REMEDIES

For insect bites, you can either apply fresh *Aloe
vera* sap or fresh lemon balm or plantain leaves
to the wound in order to bring about relief. Bathe
the affected area with marigold tea, if the bite
becomes infected.

HOMEOPATHIC REMEDIES

Hypericum tincture or lotion can be applied to the
skin and may be soothing.

Ledum 30c

For insect bites with a lot of swelling. Discomfort
eased when bathing in cold water or a cold compress applied. May prevent mosquito bites in
people who are often bitten (for prevention: 1
tablet daily for a maximum of 14 days). Also useful
in animal bites and all puncture wounds.

Apis 30c

For burning of surrounding area. Swelling often
marked. Worse for heat.

DOSAGE 1 tablet every 30 minutes (every 15 minutes for a severe reaction). Maximum six doses.

AROMATHERAPY

Put a drop of undiluted lavender directly onto the
area of skin affected by the bite.

KITCHEN MEDICINE

A real old wives' reme-
dy if you are out in the
countryside is to chew
a mouthful of plantain
leaves and apply the
resulting paste to the
wound. Flea bites
should be rubbed with
a slice of raw onion;
mosquito bites with
the cut end of a
clove of garlic.

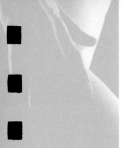

Stings

Stings, by insects and marine animals, vary in strength and seriousness, but often result in localized pain, reddening, and swelling, and sometimes in nausea, fainting, and breathing problems.

BEES

✚ CONVENTIONAL MEDICINE

If the sting is visible, remove it with tweezers. Apply a cold compress. Use calamine or antihistamine to reduce the itch, and apply insect repellent to prevent further bites.

HERBAL REMEDIES

Apply a slice of onion to bee and wasp stings, or try marigold cream or crushed plantain leaves.

Bathe the area with a marigold infusion, after removing any remaining sting.

AROMATHERAPY

Remove the sting if possible, then put 1 drop of undiluted lavender on the affected area, repeating the treatment if necessary following a plant sting (e.g. from a nettle).

❁ HOMEOPATHIC REMEDIES

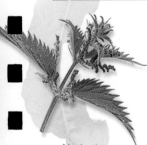

ABOVE Nettle stings can be relieved by rubbing with a dock leaf.

~ **Ledum 30c**
For insect stings where there is a lot of swelling. Discomfort eased when bathing affected area in cold water or a cold compress is applied.

~ **Apis 30c**
For burning and stinging of surrounding area. Swelling often marked. Worse for heat. Good treatment for bee and wasp stings.

DOSAGE 1 tablet every 30 minutes (every 15 minutes for a severe reaction). Maximum six doses.

KITCHEN MEDICINE

For wasp stings, make a paste of salt and vinegar, then spread over the affected area. For bee stings, use baking powder or sodium bicarbonate, mixed to a smooth paste—making sure that you remove the sting.

The traditional remedy for stinging-nettle burns is the dock leaf, but an ordinary, used teabag dipped in ice water can be equally soothing; as can a cup of nettle tea.

Caution

Wasps are the most likely to sting the inside of your mouth or throat. Sucking ice cubes will relieve the swelling, but at the slightest sign of breathing difficulties, rush to your nearest hospital.

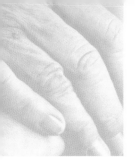

Burns

Burns are often accompanied by shock. Never, never use butter or oil on them. For small areas, run the affected part under cold water, or immerse the burned area until the pain diminishes—usually for at least 10–15 minutes.

Caution

Severe burns need urgent hospital treatment.

 CONVENTIONAL MEDICINE

Run cold water onto the burned skin until the burning sensation stops. Remove burned clothing, unless it is stuck to the burn. Cover with clean, non-fluffy material, such as a clean pillowcase, a plastic bag or plastic wrap. If the burn is extensive, located on the face, or anywhere near the mouth, seek immediate medical advice.

 HOMEOPATHIC REMEDIES

For minor burns, cool the area with cold water. Chemical burns need specialist treatment.

Arnica 30c
Initial remedy to take after any trauma.
DOSAGE 1 tablet every 15 minutes for four doses. Then try the following:

Cantharis 30c
For burn that feels as if it is raw, with severe pains. Better for cold being applied. May have blistering.
DOSAGE 1 tablet every 15 minutes for six doses, then every 4 hours. Maximum 12 doses.

KITCHEN MEDICINE

Anyone who has suffered from sunburn or serious burns, to an area greater than your hand can readily cover, should be given plenty of fluids to drink in order to prevent dehydration.

 HERBAL REMEDIES

For minor burns, apply a compress soaked in some cool chickweed, St. John's wort, marigold, or plantain infusion.

A little infused oil of St. John's wort placed on the burn, after first cooling the area under a running tap, may be soothing; fresh sap from an *Aloe vera* plant is also effective.

 AROMATHERAPY

First run the burn under freezing cold water, then immediately put some undiluted lavender oil on it.

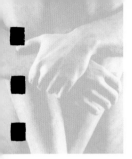

Sunburn

Sunburn is caused by ultraviolet rays and your susceptibility depends on your coloring and the amount of pigment in your skin. It is difficult to believe there is anyone unaware of the links between excessive sun exposure and skin cancer.

CONVENTIONAL MEDICINE

Find some shade and drink plenty of cold water. Sponge the sunburned skin with cold water or soak it in a cold bath. Mild burns can be soothed with calamine or an after-sun preparation.

HERBAL REMEDIES

Apply infused St. John's wort oil with a few drops of lavender oil to the sunburned area; *Aloe vera* sap is also soothing.

Drink an infusion of lime flowers, elderflowers, and yarrow in order to encourage sweating from the body.

HOMEOPATHIC REMEDIES

Belladonna 6c

For red face, very hot to touch, "could fry an egg on it." Throbbing headache, worse for light and noise. May have high fever and dilated pupils.

Glonoine 6c

For bursting headache with waves of pulsating pain. Worse during hours of sun, even if not directly exposed to it. Worse for moving. Face may be flushed or pale.

DOSAGE 1 tablet every half-hour for six doses, then every 4 hours. Maximum 4 days.

AROMATHERAPY

Add peppermint or lavender to a cool bath or, if the sunburn is quite bad, drip undiluted lavender oil on the skin after a cool bath, repeating every 2–3 hours if necessary. If the sunburned area is tender to touch, apply the oils in a water spray. Avoid peppermint if you have a gallbladder or liver problem.

KITCHEN MEDICINE

Relieve mild to moderate sunburn by putting three or four chamomile teabags into a tepid bath and soaking for 15 minutes. A mixture of one part olive oil and two parts cider vinegar, rubbed gently into the affected skin, will also help.

 Call the physician

For cases of severe sunburn with blisters.

Sprains

*A sprain occurs when the ligaments
surrounding and supporting a joint
are either overstretched or torn, most
commonly in the ankle or wrist.*

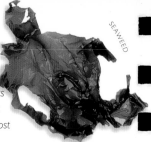

SEAWEED

KITCHEN MEDICINE

An ice pack applied
to the injury *(see
Nosebleeds on p.182)*
will help. Soothing
baths bring great relief:
add a heaped table-
spoon of mustard
powder or a cup of
Epsom salt. A bucket
of seawater added
to a hot bath, or a
handful of seaweed,
can also be extremely
healing for sprains.

 CONVENTIONAL MEDICINE

Apply an ice pack or cold compress as soon as possible to reduce swelling and bruising. Put on a
bandage or ace wrap to provide gentle, even pressure. Avoid using the sprained joint, and raise it in a
sling or on a footstool. Take a pain-reliever.

HOMEOPATHIC REMEDIES

❧ Arnica 30c
Take for the initial bruising.
DOSAGE I tablet every 15 minutes for four doses.
Continue if bruising is the main problem, at a dose
of I tablet twice daily. Maximum 5 days.

❧ Ledum 6c
For sprains, particularly of the ankle, when it is black
with bruising and is better for cold compresses.

❧ Rhus toxicodendron 6c
Pain worse on initial movement, improves as joint is
"warmed up" by movement. Worse in the morning
when the joint seems stiff. Better during the day
and for warm weather. Person may be restless.
DOSAGE I tablet three times daily. Maximum 2 weeks.

HERBAL REMEDIES

Use crushed cabbage leaves as a poultice on the
affected area.

Apply arnica or marigold creams, with a few
drops of lavender or thyme oil added; or use a
compress soaked in an infusion or diluted tincture
of one of these herbs.

 AROMATHERAPY

Ice the sprain to reduce any swelling, then massage
the whole area using lavender and chamomile.

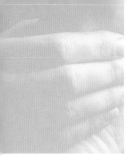

Fractures

A fracture is a broken or cracked bone, which is generally caused either by direct force (such as a blow or a kick) or by indirect force, in which case, the bone breaks at some distance from the actual point of force.

➕ CONVENTIONAL MEDICINE

Keep the fractured bone still. Discourage the injured person from drinking or eating anything, in case surgery is necessary. Support the injured part with your hands without moving it. If possible, make a sling to hold a broken arm against the body; a broken leg can be strapped to the other leg for support. Seek urgent medical attention.

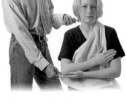

To make a sling, lay a triangular bandage with the point beyond the elbow of the injured arm.

❋ HOMEOPATHIC REMEDIES

Homeopathic remedies may assist orthodox medical treatment.

✍ Arnica 30c

Take this remedy first, for the associated bruising.

DOSAGE I tablet every 2 hours for six doses.

✍ Symphytum 6c (also called boneset/boneknit)

May help with the joining up of the broken bones. Also used when the fracture is slow to mend.

✍ Calcarea phosphorica 6c

Use if symphytum does not help.

DOSAGE I tablet twice daily. Maximum 14 days.

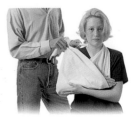

Lift the lower end of the bandage over the injured arm while the patient supports it.

▱ HERBAL REMEDIES

Drink an infusion of horsetail, alfalfa, and comfrey to encourage healing. Do not use comfrey if you are pregnant or use horsetail if you have a heart or kidney problem.

⬤ AROMATHERAPY

You cannot massage the fracture itself, so you need to work on the corresponding area (i.e. if the wrist is fractured, massage the ankle on the same side; for the shoulder, work the hip). Choose a soothing essential oil (see Stress on p.36).

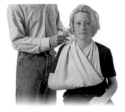

Tie the end to the neck end by the collarbone. Tuck in (or pin) the bandage by the elbow.

Nosebleeds

Nosebleeds may be caused by an illness, a blow, or by the rupture of blood vessels in the nose; dry air can cause nasal membranes to dry out and crack; and sometimes, nosebleeds occur spontaneously for no apparent reason.

KITCHEN MEDICINE

Crush a few cubes of ice and wrap them in a clean handkerchief. Place this ice pack over the top of the nose and apply pressure with thumb and forefinger on each side for at least 5–6 minutes. If bleeding persists, add 2tsp of cider vinegar to a glass of tepid water, tip the head back, and use a dropper to trickle the mixture into each nostril. Apply petroleum jelly to a dry nose to prevent bleeds.

 CONVENTIONAL MEDICINE

Sit down, leaning forward. Breathing through the mouth, pinch the soft part of the nose below the bridge. Avoid sniffing, swallowing, coughing, or spitting, which might provoke further bleeding. Use a handkerchief or cloth to mop up the blood. Release the pressure after 10 minutes. If bleeding continues, reapply pressure for another 10 minutes. After 30 minutes, if the bleeding has not stopped, seek medical advice. If the bleeding does stop, you should rest quietly for several hours and avoid sniffing or blowing. If a broken nose is suspected, keep holding the nose and get medical help.

 HOMEOPATHIC REMEDIES

For persistent nosebleeds, consult your physician.

Arnica 30c

For nosebleeds resulting from a blow to the nose. This helps stop the bleeding.

Phosphorus 30c

Often used in children. For nosebleeds for no apparent reason. Bright red blood, and nosebleeds when blowing the nose.

DOSAGE 1 tablet every 15 minutes. Maximum six doses.

 HERBAL REMEDIES

A traditional and effective herbal remedy is simply to insert a yarrow leaf in the affected nostril and then pinch the nose together gently until a blood clot forms.

Insert a small cotton swab soaked in shepherd's purse, witch hazel, lady's mantle, agrimony, or yarrow tincture into the nostril.

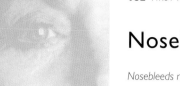

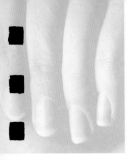

Splinters

Splinters are generally small pieces of wood or thorn that get embedded in the skin and may cause infection. Soak the affected area in hot, very soapy water before squeezing the splinter out or removing it with a sterilized needle or tweezers.

 CONVENTIONAL MEDICINE

If possible, remove the splinter with tweezers. If the splinter is deeply embedded or difficult to remove, seek medical attention. Clean the area around the splinter with soap and warm water. Check that your tetanus immunization is up to date.

 HERBAL REMEDIES

Use a little chickweed, marshmallow, or slippery-elm ointment to help draw stubborn splinters: apply the ointment, cover with a small bandage, and leave for a few hours before extracting the splinter with tweezers or a clean needle.

 AROMATHERAPY

Remove the splinter with tweezers or a sterilized needle, then apply 1 drop of undiluted lavender oil to the site.

 HOMEOPATHIC REMEDIES

Remove the splinter if at all possible. Watch for signs of infection.

🐛 **Silicea 6c**

Reputed to expel foreign material from the body. Care should be taken, as it may also aid expulsion of pins or screws used to keep a fracture in place! Has been known to irritate dental fillings. If this occurs, stop.

DOSAGE 1 tablet twice daily. Maximum 14 days.

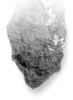
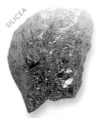

SILICEA

RIGHT Marsh-mallow ointment helps draw out splinters.

KITCHEN MEDICINE

For stubborn and difficult splinters, cover the area with a hot bread poultice, which will help to draw the splinter to the surface. Make this by putting three or four slices of bread (white, brown, or whole wheat—it makes no real difference) into a sieve. Pour over boiling water, then mash with a wooden spoon until you have a thick, hot paste. Make sure that the temperature is not too hot before applying. For really stubborn splinters, especially underneath finger- or toenails, you may need several applications.

Motion sickness

Any form of motion can cause the nausea, vomiting, and dizziness that we know as motion sickness. It is much more common in children, but adults too can suffer. There is a link between severe motion sickness in children and adult migraine.

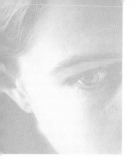

CANDIED GINGER

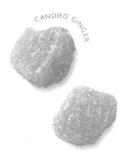

ABOVE Ginger in all its forms can alleviate nausea and sickness.

KITCHEN MEDICINE

Ginger is the king of kitchen remedies, but for maximum benefit you need to administer it before the sickness starts. Fill a thermos flask with ginger tea and, after your pre-travel mugful, sip a small cup every hour. Avoid ginger if you have gallstones For children, buy candied ginger, cut it into small cubes, and give to the youngster to nibble on every half-hour.

CONVENTIONAL MEDICINE

Symptoms can be prevented by lying flat with closed eyes. Try to avoid reading while moving. If possible, get out of the vehicle or take a break from traveling.

HOMEOPATHIC REMEDIES

Homeopathic motion-sickness pills (a combination of remedies) are available at some pharmacies

Cocculus 30c

For nausea and giddiness at even the thought of food. Lots of saliva. Giddiness better for lying down. Worse for watching moving objects, for loss of sleep, light, and noise.

Tabacum 30c

For person convinced they will die of nausea. Pale with cold sweats. Worse for opening eyes and smell of tobacco. Better in fresh cold air (on deck).

Petroleum 30c

For nausea that is worse for sitting up, noise. Better for eating. Lots of saliva.

DOSAGE I tablet every 30 minutes until improved. Maximum six doses.

HERBAL REMEDIES

Drink a cup of ginger, chamomile, black horehound, or lemon balm as tea, or use 2–3 drops of tincture on the tongue at regular intervals.

AROMATHERAPY

Put a couple of drops of ginger or peppermint oil on a handkerchief. Avoid peppermint if you have a liver or gallbladder problem and avoid ginger if you have gallstones.

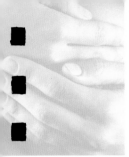

Fainting

Fainting is caused by a temporary reduction in the supply of blood to the brain. It may be due to a shock, fear or exhaustion, missed meals, excessive heat , or standing still for too long.

✚ CONVENTIONAL MEDICINE

Call 911 and encourage the person to lie down with legs raised about 6in, until he or she feels completely better. Check for injuries, such as bruising or cuts. Make a note of the events that occurred before, during, and after the faint (useful information for the physician) and encourage the patient to have a medical check-up.

❊ HOMEOPATHIC REMEDIES

Carbo vegetabilis 6c
For chilly person, who collapses with cold sweats. Wants air and to be fanned. Fainting from too much food.

Phosphorus 6c
For open, lively, and artistic person. Sympathetic and sensitive to external impressions. Fainting from hunger.

Ignatia 6c
For fainting from emotional shock. Person is grief-stricken, sighing. Intolerant of tobacco. Lump in throat, as if about to cry.
DOSAGE 1 tablet every 10 minutes. Maximum 12 tablets. Crush tablet and place powder on the tongue.

⬤ AROMATHERAPY

Loosen all clothing, then waft some rosemary or basil oil under the nose. Avoid these oils if the person is pregnant.

HERBAL REMEDIES

Sniff camphor or tea-tree oil.
Drink chamomile or betony tea to help recovery, once consciousness is regained.

KITCHEN MEDICINE

A cup of hot green or Indian tea should be sipped once the fainting has passed. And inhaling the aroma from a small piece of crushed horseradish is a good substitute for old-fashioned smelling salts.

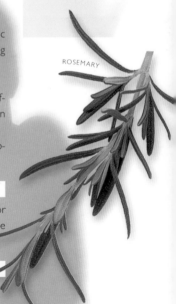

ROSEMARY

Herbal remedies
basic methods

Although it is possible to buy many herbal remedies commercially, it is often cheaper to make your own at home and create just the amount you need. All quantities given throughout the herbal sections refer to dried herbs, rather than fresh.

MAKING A COMPRESS

A compress (either hot or cold) is an effective way of applying a herbal remedy directly to the site of an inflammation or skin wound in order to speed up the healing process. Soak a clean linen or cotton cloth, or a pad of cotton gauze, in a hot infusion or decoction (see below and p.187). Apply the compress to the affected skin while it's as hot as is bearable. To maintain its temperature, either change the compress as it cools down or cover it with plastic or waxed paper, and then with a hot-water bottle. Prepare a cold compress in the same way, but allow it to cool before applying directly to the skin.

MAKING A POULTICE

A poultice consists of a pulp made directly of herbs. It is often used to draw pus out of the skin. Mix dried herbs with a little hot water until you have a paste; or use the mushy herbs left over from a hot infusion or decoction (see below and p.187); or process fresh herbs in a blender or food processor. Sandwich the paste between two layers of gauze, then apply to the affected skin while it's as hot as is bearable, changing it or placing a hot-water bottle on top, as for a compress.

MAKING AN INFUSION

Infusions are the most versatile method of taking herbal remedies, since you can drink them as teas or tisanes (hot or cold, sweetened with a little honey, if desired); use them as a mouth-wash, gargle or eyebath (simmered to sterilize, then cooled); or add them to the bath. They are made from the flowers or leaves of the plant, which readily release their active ingredients. Warm a china or glass teapot, then add the dried herb, breaking it into small pieces if necessary. Cover with near-boiling water. Allow 1–2tsp of the herb for each cup of water. Steep for 5–10 minutes, then strain and drink. Make fresh infusions each day.

MAKING A DECOCTION

Decoctions are similar to infusions, and are used in much the same way, but involve boiling the herb to release its active ingredients. This enables woody stems, roots, bark, berries, and seeds to be used. Chop or crush the herb into an enamel, stainless-steel, or glass-lidded pan (never aluminum). Cover with cold water. Allow 1½ cups/350ml of water to ½–1tsp of herb. Bring to a boil and simmer for 10–15 minutes or until the volume is reduced by one-third. Strain and use while still hot. It is preferable to make fresh decoctions daily.

MAKING A TINCTURE

Tinctures are alcohol preparations. The alcohol dissolves most of the herb's useful ingredients and preserves the preparation. Tinctures are stronger than infusions or decoctions and are best diluted with a little water. Place some chopped or powdered herb in a container with a tightly fitting lid. Use a ratio of 1 part herb to 5 parts liquid (e.g. 1lb to 5pt, or 200g to 1liter). Make a water/alcohol mix by diluting a bottle of vodka with half its amount of water. Pour the mix over the herb. Leave for 2 weeks, shaking regularly, then strain through cheesecloth, squeezing it out well. Pour into dark glass bottles and keep well stoppered in a cool, dark place. The dosage is generally 1tsp three times a day.

MAKING A SUGAR SYRUP

Syrups are concentrated sugar preparations, which help preserve infusions and decoctions and mask the unpalatable taste of some herbs. They can make cough mixtures and herbal brews more acceptable to children. Bring some of your selected infusion or decoction to a boil with honey or sugar, using the ratio 1pt liquid to 1lb honey or sugar (500ml to 500g). Cook until the mixture turns syrupy, then store until required in a corked (not a screwtop) bottle. Because of the risk of botulism, children under two should not be given honey.

Herbs mentioned
with botanical names

COMMON NAME	Botanical name
AGRIMONY	Agrimonia eupatoria
ALEXANDRIAN SENNA	see Senna
ALFALFA	Medicago sativa
ALOE VERA	Aloe vera
AMERICAN ARBORVITAE	see Thuja
AMERICAN CRANESBILL	see Cranesbill
AMERICAN GINSENG	Panax quinquefolius
ANGELICA	Angelica archangelica
ANISE	Pimpinella anisum
ARABIAN COFFEE	see Coffee
ARNICA	Arnica montana
ASTRAGALUS	Astragalus membranaceus
BASIL	Ocimum basilicum
BAYBERRY	Myrica cerifera
BEARBERRY	Arctostaphylos uva-ursi
BENZOIN	Styrax benzoin
(FRIAR'S BALSAM—compound tincture of benzoin)	
BETONY	Stachys officinalis
BILBERRY	Vaccinium myrtillus
BIRCH	Betula pendula
BISTORT	Polygonum bistorta
BLACK COHOSH	Cimicifuga racemosa
BLACK HAW	Viburnum prunifolium
BLACK HOREHOUND	Ballota nigra
BLESSED THISTLE	see Holy Thistle
BLUE FLAG	Iris versicolor
BOGBEAN	Menyanthes trifoliata
BONESET	Eupatorium perfoliatum
BORAGE	Borago officinalis
BROAD-LEAVED DOCK	see Dock
BUCHU	Agathosma crenulata
BUCKWHEAT	Fagopyrum esculentum
	(now known as Polygonum fagopyrum)
BURDOCK	Arctium lappa
CABBAGE	Brassica oleracea
CADE OIL	see Eucalyptus
CALIFORNIAN POPPY	Eschscholzia californica
CARAWAY	Carum carvi
CARDAMOM	Elettaria cardamomum
CASCARA SAGRADA	Rhamnus purshianus
CATMINT	Nepeta cataria
CATNIP	see Catmint
CAYENNE	Capsicum frutescens
CENTAURY	Centaurium erythraea
CEYLON CINNAMON	see Cinnamon
CHAMOMILE	Matricaria recutita
CHASTEBERRY	Vitex agnus-castus
CHICKWEED	Stellaria media
CHILI	Capsicum anuum
CHILI PEPPER	see Chili
CHINESE FIGWORT	Scrophularia ningpoensis
(XUAN SHEN)	
CINNAMON	Cinnamomum zeylanicum
CLEAVERS	Galium aparine
CLOVE	Syzygium aromaticum

COMMON NAME	Botanical name
COFFEE	Coffea arabica
COLTSFOOT	Tussilago farfara
COMFREY	Symphytum officinale
COMMON BALM	see Lemon balm
COMMON BASIL	see Basil
COMMON BEARBERRY	see Bearberry
COMMON CENTAURY	see Centaury
COMMON COMFREY	see Comfrey
COMMON DANDELION	see Dandelion
COMMON FUMITORY	see Fumitory
COMMON GINGER	see Ginger
COMMON HOP	see Hops
COMMON HORSE CHESTNUT	see Horse chestnut
COMMON HOREHOUND	see White horehound
COMMON HORSETAIL	see Horsetail
COMMON HOUSE LEEK	see House leek
COMMON JUNIPER	see Juniper
COMMON MULLEIN	see Mullein
COMMON PLANTAIN	Plantago major
COMMON SAGE	see Sage
COMMON THYME	see Thyme
COMMON VALERIAN	see Valerian
COMMON WORMWOOD	see Wormwood
COMMON YARROW	see Yarrow
CORIANDER	Coriandrum sativum
CORNSILK	Zea mays
COUCHGRASS	Elymus repens
COWSLIP	Primula veris
CRAMP BARK	Viburnum opulus
CRANBERRY	Vaccinium oxycoccos
CRANESBILL	Geranium spp.
CURLED DOCK	see Yellow dock
CYPRESS	Cupressus sempervirens
DAMIANA	Turnera diffusa
DANDELION	Taraxacum officinale
DEVIL'S CLAW	Harpagophytum procumbens
DILL	Anethum graveolens
DOCK	Rumex obtusifolius
DONG QUAI	Angelica polyphorma var. sinensis
ECHINACEA	Echinacea spp.
ELDER	Sambucus nigra
ELECAMPANE	Inula helenium
ENGLISH LAVENDER	see Lavender
ENGLISH OAK	see Oak
ENGLISH PLANTAIN	Plantago lanceolata
EPHEDRA	Ephedra distachya
EUCALYPTUS	Eucalyptus globulus
EUROPEAN ELDER	see Elder
EUROPEAN WHITE BIRCH	see Birch
EUROPEAN WILD PANSY	see Heartsease
EVENING PRIMROSE	Oenothera biennis
EYEBRIGHT	Euphrasia officinalis
FALSE UNICORN ROOT	see Helonias
FENNEL	Foeniculum vulgare
FENUGREEK	Trigonella foenum graecum

COMMON NAME	Botanical name
FEVERFEW	Tanacetum parthenium
FORSYTHIA	Forsythia suspensa
FRAGRANT SUMACH	see Sweet sumach
FUMITORY	Fumaria officinalis
GARLIC	Allium sativa
GENTIAN	Gentiana lutea
GINGER	Zingiber officinale
GINSENG	Panax ginseng
GOLDENSEAL	Hydrastis canadensis
GOTU KOLA	Centella asiatica
GREATER CELANDINE	Chelidonium majus
GUM BENZOIN	see Benzoin
HEARTSEASE	Viola tricolor
HELONIAS	Chamaelirium luteum
HERB ROBERT	Geranium robertianum
HE SHOU WU/FO TI	Polygonum multiflorum
HOLY THISTLE	Cnicus benedictus
HOPS	Humulus lupulus
HORSE CHESTNUT	Aesculus hippocastanum
HORSERADISH	Armoracia rusticana
HORSETAIL	Equisetum arvense
HOUSE LEEK	Sempervivum tectorum
HYSSOP	Hyssopus officinalis
ITALIAN CYPRESS	see Cypress
JASMINE	Jasminum officinale
JUNIPER	Juniperus communis
KELP	Fucus versiculosus
KING'S CLOVER	see Sweet clover
KOREAN GINSENG	see Ginseng
LADY'S MANTLE	Alchemilla vulgaris
LARGE CRANBERRY	see Cranberry
LAVENDER	Lavandula angustifolia
LEMON BALM	Melissa officinalis
LESSER CELANDINE	see Pilewort
LICORICE	Glycyrrhiza glabra
LIME FLOWERS	Tilia cordata
LOVAGE	Levisticum officinale
MAD-DOG SKULLCAP	see Skullcap
MARIGOLD	Calendula officinalis
MARJORAM	Origanum majorana
MARSHMALLOW	Althaea officinalis
MEADOWSWEET	Filipendula ulmaria
MOTHERWORT	Leonurus cardiaca
MUGWORT	Artemisia vulgaris
MULLEIN	Verbascum thapsus
MYRRH	Commiphora molmol
NARROW-LEAVED PLANTAIN	see English Plantain
NUTMEG	Myristica fragrans
OAK	Quercus robur
OATS	Avena sativa
ONION	Allium cepa
PAPAYA	Carica papaya
PARSLEY	Petroselinum crispum
PASSION FLOWER	Passiflora incarnata
PEPPERMINT	Mentha x piperita
PILEWORT	Ranunculus ficaria
PINE	Pinus sylvestris
POET'S JESSAMINE	see Jasmine
POTENTILLA	Potentilla anserina
POT MARIGOLD	see Marigold
PSYLLIUM	Plantago psyllium
PURPLE CONE FLOWER	see Echinacea
RASPBERRY	Rubus idaeus
RED CLOVER	Trifolium pratense
RED RASPBERRY	see Raspberry
REISHI	Ganoderma lucidum
ROSE	Rosa spp.
ROSEMARY	Rosmarinus officinalis

COMMON NAME	Botanical name
SAGE	Salvia officinalis
ST. JOHN'S WORT	Hypericum perforatum
SANDALWOOD	Santalum album
SANICLE	Sanicula europaea
SCOTS PINE	see Pine
SELF-HEAL	Prunella vulgaris
SENNA	Senna alexandrina
SHEPHERD'S PURSE	Capsella bursa-pastoris
SHIITAKE MUSHROOM	Lentinus edodes
SIBERIAN GINSENG	Eleutherococcus senticosus
SKULLCAP	Scutellaria lateriflora
SLIPPERY ELM	Ulmus rubra
SOAPWORT	Saponaria oficinalis
STINGING NETTLE	Urtica dioica
SWEET CLOVER	Melilotus officinalis
SWEET MARJORAM	see Marjoram
SWEET SUMACH	Rhus aromatica
SWEET VIOLET	see Violet
TABASCO PEPPER	see Cayenne
TANGERINE	Citrus reticulata
TEA	Camellia sinensis
TEA TREE	Melaleuca alternifolia
THUJA	Thuja occidentalis
THYME	Thymus vulgaris
TORMENTIL	Potentilla erecta
TURNIP	Brassica 'Rapifero Group'
VALERIAN	Valeriana officinalis
VERVAIN	Verbena officinalis
VIOLET	Viola odorata
WHITE HOREHOUND	Marrubium vulgare
WHITE SANDALWOOD	see Sandalwood
WILD BLACK CHERRY	see Wild cherry
WILD CHERRY	Prunus serotina
WILD INDIGO	Baptisia tinctoria
WILD LETTUCE	Lactuca virosa
WILD PASSION FLOWER	see Passion flower
WILD YAM	Dioscorea villosa
WINTERGREEN	Gaultheria procumbens
WITCH HAZEL	Hamamelis virginiana
WORMWOOD	Artemisia absintheum
WOUNDWORT	Stachys palustris
YARROW	Achillea millefolium
YELLOW DOCK	Rumex crispus
YELLOW GENTIAN	see Gentian

Most useful
herbal remedies

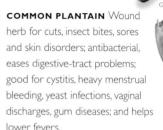

GARLIC

AGRIMONY Soothes digestive problems; helps treat cuts and scrapes, skin problems, minor eye problems, sore throats, and congestion of the respiratory tract.

ALOE VERA Effective for skin problems, minor cuts and burns, insect bites, digestive problems; acts as an appetite stimulant and tonic. Avoid if you are pregnant or have a bowel disorder. Do not give to children under 12.

BETONY Eases anxiety and stress; treats headaches, cuts and bruises, mouth and gum disorders, sore throats; encourages contractions in childbirth; acts as a digestive stimulant and a circulatory tonic.

CHAMOMILE Beneficial for digestive problems, poor appetite, insomnia, nervous tension and anxiety, mouth inflammations and sore throats, nasal congestion, minor eye problems, eczema and skin problems, asthma and hay fever; homeopathic dilutions are used for colic, restlessness, and teething problems in babies and toddlers.

COMMON PLANTAIN Wound herb for cuts, insect bites, sores and skin disorders; antibacterial, eases digestive-tract problems; good for cystitis, heavy menstrual bleeding, yeast infections, vaginal discharges, gum diseases; and helps lower fevers.

ECHINACEA Antibacterial, antiviral, and antifungal for a range of infections (including colds/flu), skin problems, sore throats, kidney infections. Avoid if you are pregnant or have a specific disorder of the immune system.

ELDER Flowers are useful for colds, flu, congestion, hay fever, fevers and inflammation; leaves can be used in ointments for bruises and sores.

GARLIC Antibacterial, antifungal, and antiseptic; lowers blood cholesterol levels and helps combat candidiasis and respiratory infections; boosts the immune system.

GINGER Warming for chills and colds; combats nausea and vomiting; beneficial for digestive problems; acts as a circulatory stimulant. Avoid if you have gallstones.

LAVENDER Sedative for migraines, headaches, insomnia, and stress; good for digestive upsets; use externally on burns, scrapes, and sunburn.

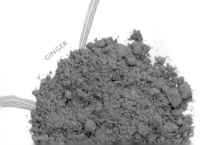

GINGER

LEMON BALM Calming for digestive upsets and nervous problems; antidepressive; antibacterial—useful for infections and fevers; use externally to treat wounds and insect bites, and as an effective insect repellent.

MARIGOLD Good in creams for cuts, grazes, fungal infections, eczema, and many other skin problems; acts as a digestive stimulant and as a menstrual regulator; helps lower fevers; beneficial for gum disease and swollen glands.

MARSHMALLOW Soothing for digestive tract inflammations and ulcers, urinary inflammations, coughs, congestion; use externally for skin sores, boils, abscesses, and for drawing splinters and pus.

MEADOWSWEET Calming antacid for digestive upsets; good for arthritic and rheumatic disorders; antiseptic and cooling. Do not use if you are sensitive to aspirin.

ROSEMARY Stimulating and restorative for nervous exhaustion and depression; beneficial for headaches, migraine, digestive problems; use externally for arthritic and rheumatic pains. Avoid if you are pregnant or if you are breastfeeding.

ST. JOHN'S WORT Antidepressive, sedative, restorative for the nervous system; useful in anxiety, nervous tension, depression, neuralgia, post-operative pain, period pain; antiseptic and soothing—useful topically for burns, skin sores, cuts, and scrapes.

TEA TREE Antiseptic, antifungal; useful for all infections, including yeast infections, athlete's foot, ringworm, septicemia, tooth and gum infections and abscesses, warts, cold sores, acne, insect stings and bites.

THYME Respiratory antiseptic and expectorant for coughs and bronchitis; acts as a digestive stimulant—warming for both chills and diarrhea; the oil is antiseptic, useful as a wound herb and in cases of infection.

VERVAIN Relaxing nervine for depression and tension; acts as a digestive and liver stimulant; used in childbirth to ease labor pains; used topically for nerve pains (neuralgia).

YARROW Used in fevers and to dilate peripheral blood vessels; acts as a wound herb, digestive tonic, and is helpful for both urinary and menstrual irregularities.

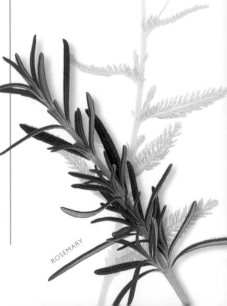

ROSEMARY

Most useful conventional remedies

ACETAMINOPHEN (e.g. Tylenol) A pain killer used to treat headaches, sprains, and fever. Many over-the-counter medications combine acetaminophen with other drugs, such as codeine phosphate and caffeine, to enhance their effect. Codeine phosphate may cause constipation. Unlike aspirin, acetaminophen does not cause gastrointestinal bleeding. *Avoid if you have liver problems.*

ANTACIDS Relieve indigestion and heartburn. Magnesium-based antacids (e.g. Milk of Magnesia) may cause diarrhea; those containing aluminum (Alu-Cap) or calcium (Tums) may cause constipation. Some formulas include both aluminum and magnesium (Maalox). Others contain dimethicone to relieve gas (Gas-X).

ANTIHISTAMINES Relieve hay fever symptoms. Over-the-counter versions usually cause drowsiness.

Prescription antihistamines, such as loratadine (Claritin), may not.

BECLOMETHASONE DIPROPRIONATE (Beconase) A prescription steroid nasal spray that relieves long-term hay fever symptoms, such as nasal congestion or runny nose. If it causes dryness and crusting, consult your doctor for an alternative medication.

BENZOCAINE (e.g. Chloraseptic) A local anesthetic available in either lozenge or spray form; relieves the pain of sore throats.

CALAMINE Found in many creams and lotions used to treat itchy skin.

CHLORPHENIRAMINE MALEATE TABLETS (e.g. Chlor-Trimetron) Controls hay fever symptoms and itchy skin; prevents jet lag and motion sickness. Like other non-prescription antihistamines, causes drowsiness.

CIMETIDINE (Tagamet) May relieve indigestion that does not respond to an antacid. *Avoid in pregnancy.*

CLOTRIMAZOLE (e.g. Gyne-Lotrimin) An antifungal agent available in creams and suppositories for the relief of yeast infections. May cause stinging (if so, consult your doctor for an alternative medication).

EMOLLIENTS (e.g. petroleum jelly or lanolin) Help alleviate dry skin. Almond oil can be used to soften ear wax prior to syringing.

FLUCONAZOLE (Diflucan) A prescription tablet alternative to creams/suppositories for the treatment of vaginal yeast infections. Only one tablet is usually needed in order to clear up symptoms. *Avoid in pregnancy.*

HYDROCORTISONE ACETATE 0.5–1% A mild steroid cream that is useful for skin irritation, such as mild eczema.

IBUPROFEN (e.g. Advil, Motrin) A pain killer, especially helpful in cases of inflammation—e.g. sprains, backache, or swollen joints. *Avoid if you have asthma or stomach ulcers. Avoid in pregnancy.*

LOPERAMIDE (Imodium A-D) or **BISMUTH SUBSALICYLATE** (Pepto-Bismol) Useful in controlling routine cases of diarrhea.

METHOL SALICYLATE (e.g. Icy Hot, Bengay) Sprayed or rubbed onto the skin, it produces heat or cold to ease a sprained joint/muscle ache.

MICONAZOLE (e.g. Micotin) A spray used to relieve fungal skin infections, such as athlete's foot. Miconazole gel is available for treating oral yeast infections (thrush). *Avoid oral treatment in pregnancy.*

PSYLLIUM (e.g. Metamucil) Useful for cases of constipation that do not seem to respond to dietary change/exercise.

CHILDREN'S REMEDIES

CHLORPHENIRAMINE MALEATE LIQUID (e.g. Chlor-Trimetron) Eases itchy skin and hay fever symptoms.

DIMETHICONE (e.g. Mylicon) Helps relieve infantile colic.

MINERAL OIL Softens cradle cap.

Also **IBUPROFEN** (e.g. Motrin) and **ACETAMINOPHEN** (e.g. Tylenol), as above. Because of the risk of Reye's syndrome, do not give aspirin to children under 16.

SYMPTOMS THAT REQUIRE URGENT MEDICAL ATTENTION

- Severe, crushing chest pain
- Difficulty breathing
- Fever above 103°F/39.5°C
- Vomiting with blood or for more than 24 hours, or prolonged diarrhea
- Loss of consciousness for more than 2 minutes
- Unexplained confused behavior
- Unexplained lethargy or weakness in a child
- Convulsions
- Severe headache, that develops very suddenly or is associated with a fever and possibly with a rash
- Difficulty swallowing saliva
- Severe abdominal pain
- Painful urination with back pain
- Uncontrollable bleeding
- Nosebleed for more than 30 minutes, despite first-aid measures
- An object, such as a bead, up the nose of a child
- Bee sting near or in the mouth
- Swallowed detergents or poisons
- Eye injury or chemicals in the eye

Homeopathy

N early 200 years ago **Samuel Hahnemann found that a medicine that causes symptoms in a well person could, in small doses, help cure the same symptoms in a sick person. In homeopathy, a patient's symptoms are matched with those associated with a particular remedy. Anything that makes the symptoms better or worse is used as a guide to individualizing the patient's symptom picture and selecting the right remedy.**

Homeopathy has many remedies, each associated with numerous symptoms. For most ailments in this book, you'll find a sampling of the homeopathic remedies commonly used to treat them, along with important symptoms associated with each remedy. Try the remedy that best matches your symptoms. If the symptoms change, consult the list again, or see a qualified homeopath.

Homeopathic remedies are repeatedly diluted in alcohol. The more diluted a remedy is, the greater its potency. A remedy labeled 6X (meaning that it has been diluted six times by a factor of 10) is weaker than a 30C remedy (diluted 30 times by a factor of 100). Remedies are usually sold in 6c or 30c potency, with lower potencies used when the remedy's accuracy is less certain. Homeopathic remedies come in pellets, tablets, liquids, and topical creams. A dose is usually one tablet, two to four pellets, or 5 to 15 drops.

BELOW Homeopathic remedies are usually kept in dark glass bottles and stored away from strong-smelling items.

Store remedies in a cool, dry place. Tip pellets or tablets into the bottle cap, then into your mouth, without touching them. Remedies should be dissolved under the tongue, not swallowed. Don't eat anything strong-tasting before taking a remedy, and don't eat or drink for 10 minutes before or after; avoid mint and coffee. Do not use during the first three months of pregnancy; seek the advice of a qualified homeopath.

Most useful homeopathic remedies

ARGENTUM NITRICUM For anxiety, chronic fatigue syndrome, depression, gastritis, IBS, laryngitis.

ARSENICUM ALBUM For diarrhea and vomiting, food poisoning, gastritis, peptic ulcers, eczema, psoriasis, hay fever, asthma.

BELLADONNA For earache, fever, tonsillitis, arthritis, German measles, scarlet fever.

BRYONIA For gastritis, indigestion, chest infections, sciatica, headache.

CHAMOMILLA For earache, teething, colic, cough, painful periods, toothache.

GELSEMIUM For fear of dentist/driving test, anxiety symptoms generally, flu, diarrhea, chronic fatigue syndrome.

HEPAR SULPHURIS For abscesses, acne, sore throat, coughs and bronchitis, earache.

IGNATIA For grief, cough, depression, headache.

IPECACUANHA For asthma, cough, nausea in pregnancy.

LACHESIS For asthma, flushes and menopausal problems, heavy periods, sore throats.

LYCOPODIUM For bowel problems, bloating, IBS, heartburn, migraine, urinary infection, premature baldness.

MERCURIUS For mouth ulcers, colds, sore throat, colitis, ear infections, ulcerative colitis.

NATRUM MURIATICUM For mouth ulcers, cold sores, asthma, eczema, psoriasis, IBS, headaches, PMS.

NUX VOMICA For stress, overwork, fatigue, insomnia, hay fever, asthma, colic, headaches, peptic ulcers.

PHOSPHORUS For peptic ulcers, gastritis, colitis, coughs and bronchitis, nosebleeds.

PULSATILLA For pregnancy sickness, breech presentations, cystitis, postnatal depression, period problems, hay fever, conjunctivitis, recurrent ear infections, IBS, bedwetting.

RHUS TOXICODENDRON For chicken pox, shingles, arthritis, rheumatism, eczema, sprains.

SEPIA For depression, fatigue, cystitis, PMS, back pain, nausea in pregnancy, warts, ringworm.

STAPHYSAGRIA For depression, cystitis related to intercourse, PMS, psoriasis (particularly after grief), warts, pain in surgical wounds.

SULPHUR For abscesses, acne, eczema, asthma, dandruff, menopausal flushes, migraine, arthritis, tonsillitis.

Aromatherapy

LAVENDER

ESSENTIAL OILS

Essential oils are extracted from the leaves, fruit, flowers, bark, roots, and wood of plants and trees and are absorbed by the body during aromatherapy, either through inhalation or the pores of the skin.

Caution

Never ingest essential oils or apply them undiluted to the skin (unless it's specifically suggested in the text), as they can cause irritation.

COMPRESSES

Add 4–6 drops of essential oil to a bowl of warm water and mix well. Soak the compress, then squeeze out the excess water (but do not wring). Apply to the affected area. If possible, wrap in plastic wrap followed by a warm towel. Keep covered for at least 2 hours (preferably overnight).

BASE/CARRIER OILS

For direct skin application, mix essential oils with a base, or carrier, oil. This enables them to penetrate the skin without causing irritation or burning. Any of the light vegetable-based oils that you ingest can also be applied to your skin.

MASSAGE OILS

To make a massage oil, add 2 drops of essential oil to 1tsp of carrier oil, or to 1tsp of aqueous cream or lotion. For a child, add 1 drop of essential oil to 2tsp of either carrier oil or cream.

STEAM INHALATIONS

Add 4–6 drops of essential oil to a bowl of hot water. Bend over the bowl, cover your head with a towel, and inhale the steam. This treatment is not suitable for asthmatics or small children. Alternatively, put 1–2 drops of oil on a handkerchief or pillow; or run hot water into the bath and sit in the steamy bathroom with a child.

BATHING WITH OILS

Run the bath, then add 4–6 drops of oil for adults and 1–2 drops for children (or mix with a carrier oil or milk first). Agitate the water, then soak for at least 20 minutes. Follow the same process for foot, hand and sitz baths.

VAPORIZERS

Never allow your burner to run dry or leave it unattended, as some essential oils are highly flammable. Put 1–2 drops of oil into the vaporizer and heat for 15–20 minutes. Then turn the vaporizer off, or blow out the candle. The effects will last for 4–6 hours. Alternatively, soak a piece of cotton in 1–2 drops of oil and place behind a warm radiator.

SPRAYS

Put 10–15 drops of essential oil into 2pt/1 liter of water, then spray lightly over the area. This is very useful if the area is too painful to be touched.

Most useful aromatherapeutic oils

BASIL Mind-clearing and focusing; helps clear the sinuses. Avoid if pregnant.

CLOVE Good for toothache; in a burner at festive occasions, used with orange, pine, and/or cinnamon.

EUCALYPTUS Beneficial for cold, flu, and sinus problems. Avoid if you have digestive problems or liver disease. Do not give to babies and small children.

FRANKINCENSE Soothing to the emotions; slows and deepens breathing; good for asthmatics.

GERANIUM Beneficial for all women's problems, (PMS and the menopause).

GINGER Warming to the muscles; beneficial for digestive disorders; good for all nausea. Do not use if you have gallstones.

JASMINE Eases labor pains; useful for postnatal blues. Do not give to babies or small children.

JUNIPER Detoxifying, both mentally and physically. Avoid if pregnant or if you have a kidney problem.

LAVENDER Calming, soothing; useful for burns and insomnia.

LEMON Good for treating both warts and verrucae.

LEMON GRASS Builds the body's resistance to fatigue; good in a foot bath for tired, restless legs; an effective insect repellent.

MANDARIN Safe and gentle, relaxing for everyone.

NEROLI The best oil for stress-related problems.

ORANGE A sunny, cheering oil—uplifting and joyful.

PETITGRAIN Good for stress conditions, where neroli is indicated but is unaffordable.

ROMAN CHAMOMILE I drop in a bath soothes a cranky child at bedtime; beneficial for skin irritations; good in a tea for digestive disorders.

ROSE The ultimate feminine oil for menstrual disruption; beneficial for emotional stress and grief.

SANDALWOOD Soothing to the skin and the emotions; good for massaging (mixed with a carrier oil or lotion) in the throat area. Do not use if you have a kidney problem.

TEA TREE Antiviral, antifungal, and antibacterial; good for warts, verrucae, and athlete's foot; boosts the immune system.

YLANG YLANG Antidepressant—a heady oil, purportedly an aphrodisiac.

EUCALYPTUS

Most useful healing foods

CARROT

APPLES Good for the heart; protective against pollution; lower cholesterol; good for food poisoning and for gastroenteritis; antibacterial and antiviral; their fiber helps digestion.

ARTICHOKES (GLOBE) Good for liver complaints, biliousness, hepatitis, and gallstones; lower cholesterol; relieve fluid retention; excellent for rheumatism, arthritis, and gout.

AVOCADOS Ideal convalescing food; good for stress and sexual problems; excellent for skin conditions; powerfully antioxidant and protective against heart disease and cancers; contain a valuable antibacterial and antifungal chemical.

BANANAS Excellent for the physically active and for anyone taking diuretics; good for PMS; very healing for the whole digestive tract; good for both constipation and diarrhea.

APPLE

AVOCADO

BANANA

CABBAGE Use cabbage juice for peptic ulcers; cabbage leaves as compresses for painful joints; cabbage soup for chest infections; the dark green leaves for anemia. Cabbage and all its relatives are protectors against a whole range of cancers.

CARROTS Good for the eyes; useful puréed to treat infant diarrhea; excellent for liver problems; great for healthy skin; protective against heart disease and lung cancer.

GARLIC The king of healing plants— antibacterial, antifungal, and good for everything from bronchitis to athlete's foot; protective against food poisoning; lowers cholesterol and blood pressure; improves circulation.

KIWI FRUIT Good for blood pressure, digestive problems, chronic fatigue, and heart problems.

LEEKS Beneficial for all breathing problems; cleansing and diuretic; excellent for gout, arthritis, and for rheumatism.

LEGUMES (DRIED PEAS, BEANS AND LENTILS) Protective against heart disease and cancers (especially of the bowel); excellent for constipation, fatigue, chronic fatigue syndrome, and diabetes.

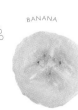

LEMONS, ORANGES, AND GRAPEFRUITS Citrus fruit are extremely rich in vitamin C and the protective bioflavonoids; strengthen natural immunity; valuable in the treatment of coughs, colds, and flu.

NUTS The healing plants and trees of tomorrow and densely full of nutrients—minerals like selenium, zinc, iron, lots of protein, healthy oils, and the B vitamins. Fresh, unsalted nuts should form a daily part of everyone's diet.

OATS Contain a cornucopia of nutrients; the best anticonstipation food; also lower cholesterol; help control blood pressure; have a calming effect on the mind and a healing effect on the stomach.

OLIVE OIL (EXTRA-VIRGIN) A remarkable food/medicine—lowers cholesterol; protects against cell damage; increases the level of the healthy blood fats that scavenge bad fats from the arteries; good for liver and gallbladder problems; protective against arthritis, senility, and even against some cancers.

ONIONS From the same family as leeks and garlic; important in the treatment of all chest infections; should be eaten by anyone who has high blood pressure, raised cholesterol, or heart disease; an excellent food for anemia, asthma, urinary infections— and even for helping with hangovers.

PINEAPPLES Like the other tropical fruits, such as mangoes and papayas, much underrated for its health benefits; ideal for sore throats, joint diseases, digestive problems, and all muscular injuries.

RICE Perfect food for convalescents, those with digestive problems, stress, and exhaustion. Brown rice is also important in the treatment of circulatory disorders. Plain boiled rice lowers cholesterol and is ideal as a treatment for diarrhea.

WATERCRESS A great protector against cancer; powerfully antibiotic, without killing off the natural bacteria; helps with urinary infections; a good stimulant of the thyroid gland.

WHEAT Highly protective against bowel disease, high blood pressure, constipation, and stress-related illnesses. Sprouted wheat seeds help in the fight against cancer. Bread can also be used as a hot poultice for boils, abscesses, and splinters.

YOGURT (LIVE) Protective against stomach infections, food poisoning, and constipation; boosts the immune system and should be eaten by those with viral or bacterial illnesses; protective against yeast and other fungal infections.

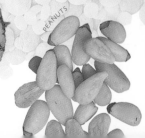

PEANUTS

PINEAPPLE

Food combining:
the Hay diet

There are many misconceptions surrounding the food combining, or Hay, diet. It is not the panacea for all ills, but it can be very beneficial for people with digestive complaints. Try it for a couple of weeks and see if it suits you—a bonus is that anyone who is overweight will certainly lose a few pounds.

The only rule that really matters is not combining starch foods and protein foods in the same meal. For example: no meat (protein) and potatoes (starch); no pasta (starch) and cheese (protein). Allow 3 hours between meals and if you want to snack, choose neutral foods, which can be eaten with starch or protein.

PROTEIN FOODS	STARCH FOODS
meat	potatoes and yams
poultry	corn
game	bread and flour
fish and shellfish	oats, wheat, and barley
eggs	rice
fruit (except those listed in the starch group)	millet and rye
peanuts	buckwheat
soybeans	pasta
tofu	very sweet fruit, such as ripe pears
milk	bananas
yogurt	papaya and mangoes
all cheese (except cream cheese and ricotta)	sweet grapes
wine and cider	beer

NEUTRAL FOODS

all vegetables (except those listed in the starch group)	beans and chickpeas (but not soybeans)
all nuts (except peanuts)	all seeds and sprouted seeds
butter and cream	herbs and spices
cream cheese and ricotta	raisins and golden raisins
egg yolk	honey and maple syrup
olive, sesame and sunflower oils	(yogurt and milk have a very low protein content, so they can be used in tiny
lentils and split peas	amounts with starch foods)

The exclusion diet

If you have a "food intolerance," try this exclusion diet for a couple of weeks. If it does not help, seek professional help. If it does help, start adding foods back one at a time to see which, if any, causes your symptoms. Exclude any culprit foods for a few months, then try them again, but any long-term removal of major food groups should only be done under professional guidance. During the first 2 weeks of the diet follow this chart to see which foods you may, and may not, eat.

FOOD	NOT ALLOWED	ALLOWED
MEAT	preserved meats, bacon, sausages, all processed meat products	all other meats
FISH	smoked fish, shellfish	white fish
VEGETABLES	potatoes, onions, corn, eggplants, bell peppers, chilis, tomatoes	all other vegetables, salads, legumes, rutabagas, parsnips
FRUIT	citrus fruits (e.g. oranges, grapefruit)	all other fruit (e.g. apples, bananas, pears)
CEREALS	wheat, oats, barley, rye, corn	rice, ground rice, rice flakes, rice flour, sago, rice breakfast cereals, tapioca, millet, buckwheat, rice cakes
COOKING OILS	corn oil, vegetable oil	sunflower oil, soy oil, safflower oil, olive oil
DAIRY PRODUCTS	cow's milk, butter, most margarines, cow's milk yogurt and cheese, eggs	goat, sheep, and soy milk and products made from them, dairy and trans fat-free margarines
BEVERAGES	tea, coffee (beans, instant, and decaffeinated), fruit smoothies, orange juice, grapefruit juice, alcohol, and tap water	herbal teas (e.g. chamomile), fresh fruit juices (e.g. apple, pineapple), pure tomato juice (without additives), mineral, distilled, or de-ionized water
MISCELLANEOUS	chocolates, yeast, yeast extracts, artificial preservatives, colorings and flavorings, monosodium glutamate, all artificial sweeteners	carob, sea salt, herbs, spices, and small amounts of sugar or honey

After 2 weeks introduce other foods in this order: tap water, potatoes, cow's milk, yeast, tea, rye, butter, onions, eggs, porridge oats, coffee, chocolate, barley, citrus fruits, corn, cow's milk cheese, white wine, shellfish, natural cow's milk yogurt, vinegar, wheat, and nuts.

Home medicine chest

Every medicine chest needs the normal range of bandages, including adhesive ones, safety pins, antiseptic, tweezers, and scissors, together with a supply of proprietary pain-relievers, antidiarrheals, and so on. However, the home medicine chest recommended here includes other natural ingredients, as powerful aids to the safe treatment of most minor ailments.

CONVENTIONAL REMEDIES

- Acetaminophen
- Calamine lotion
- Chlorpheniramine maleate
- Clotrimazole cream
- Hydrocortisone 1% cream
- Ibuprofen
- Oral rehydration liquids or powders (for reconstitution in case of diarrhea)

HERBAL REMEDIES

- A potted *Aloe vera* plant to grow on a sunny windowsill
- Arnica cream
- Chamomile flowers—loose or in teabags
- Chickweed cream
- Echinacea capsules or tincture
- Lavender oil
- Marigold cream
- Meadowsweet tincture
- Myrrh tincture
- Slippery-elm tablets
- Tea-tree oil
- Distilled witch hazel (or alternatively witch-hazel tincture)

HOMEOPATHIC REMEDIES

All at 6c potency and 30c potency.

- Aconite
- Arnica
- Apis
- Belladonna
- Bellis perennis
- Cantharis
- Hypercal ointment
- Hypericum
- Ledum
- Rhus toxicodendrum
- Silicea
- Symphytum
- Urtica urens

AROMATHERAPY OILS

It is not worth storing large quantities of essential oils, as they have a shelf-life of only 1–2 years, so unless you are going to use them regularly, do not keep a large stock of them in your medicine chest. Buy oils that have a multitude of uses for you and your family, such as the ones listed below, or oils to help specific ailments, as suggested throughout the book.

- Eucalyptus
- Lavender
- Tea tree

KITCHEN REMEDIES

- Baking soda
- Cider vinegar
- Cinnamon
- Cloves
- Epsom salt
- Garlic (fresh)
- Ginger root
- Horseradish
- Mustard powder
- Organic honey
- Sage (either a plant or dried)
- Teabags

LEFT Treat minor ailments from your home medicine chest.

Useful addresses

AROMATHERAPY

Europe

ACADEMY OF AROMATHERAPY
AND MASSAGE
50 Cow Wynd
Falkirk
Stirlingshire FK1 1PU
Great Britain
Tel: 44 1324 612658

INTERNATIONAL FEDERATION
OF AROMATHERAPISTS
Stamford House
2–4 Chiswick High Road
London W4 1TH
Great Britain
Tel: 44 208 742 2605
Fax: 44 208 742 2606

INTERNATIONAL SOCIETY
OF PROFESSIONAL
AROMATHERAPISTS
ISPA House
82 Ashby Road
Hinckley
Leics OE10 1SN
Great Britain
Tel: 44 1455 637987
Fax: 44 1455 890956

TISSERAND INSTITUTE
65 Church Road
Hove
East Sussex BN3 2BD
Great Britain
Tel: 44 1273 206640
Fax: 44 1273 329811

North America

AMERICAN ALLIANCE
OF AROMATHERAPY
PO Box 750428
Petaluma
California 94975-0428
USA
Tel: 1 707 778 6762
Fax: 1 707 769 0868

AMERICAN AROMATHERAPY
ASSOCIATION
PO Box 3679
South Pasadena
California 91031
USA
Tel: 1 818 457 1742

NATIONAL ASSOCIATION OF
HOLISTIC AROMATHERAPY
PO Box 17622
Boulder
Colorado 80308-0622
USA
Tel: 1 303 258 3791

CONVENTIONAL MEDICINE

Australasia

SKIN AND PSORIASIS
FOUNDATION
OF VICTORIA
PO Box 228
Collins Street
PO 3000
Melbourne 671962
Victoria
Australia

Europe

ARTHRITIS AND RHEUMATISM
COUNCIL FOR RESEARCH
Copeman House
St Mary's Court
St Mary's Gate
Chesterfield S41 7TD
Great Britain
Tel: 44 1246 558033

BRITISH MIGRAINE ASSOCIATION
178a High Road
Byfleet
West Byfleet
Surrey KT14 7ED
Great Britain
Tel: 44 1932 352468

HERPES ASSOCIATION
41 North Road
London N7 9DP
Great Britain
Tel: 44 207 607 9661
(Helpline: 44 207 609 9061)

MEDIC ALERT FOUNDATION
12 Bridge Wharf
156 Caledonian Road
London N1 9UU
Great Britain
Tel: 44 207 833 3034

NATIONAL ASTHMA CAMPAIGN
Providence House
Providence Place
London N1 0NT
Great Britain
Tel: 44 207 226 2260

NATIONAL BACK PAIN ASSOCIATION
16 Elmtree Road
Teddington
Middlesex TW11 8ST
Great Britain
Tel: 44 208 977 5474

WOMEN'S HEALTH CONCERN
83 Earls Court Road
London W8 6EF
Great Britain
Tel: 44 207 938 3932

North America

AMERICAN ACADEMY OF ALLERGY,
ASTHMA AND IMMUNOLOGY
611 East Wells Street
Milwaukee, Wisconsin 53202
USA
Tel: 1 800 822 2762

AMERICAN ASSOCIATION FOR
CHRONIC FATIGUE SYNDROME
c/o Harborview Medical Center
325 Ninth Avenue
Box 359780
Seattle, Washington 98104
USA
Tel: 1 206 521 1932

AMERICAN CHRONIC PAIN
ASSOCIATION
P.O. Box 850
Rocklin, California 95677
USA
Tel: 1 916 632 0922

AMERICAN HEART ASSOCIATION
7272 Greenville Avenue
Dallas, Texas 75231
USA
Tel: 1 800 242 8721

ARTHRITIS FOUNDATION
1330 West Peachtree Street
Atlanta, Georgia 30309
USA
Tel: 1 800 283-7800

BACK PAIN HOTLINE
Texas Back Institute
6300 West Parker Road
Plano, Texas 75093
USA
Tel: 1 800 247 2225

NATIONAL HEADACHE
FOUNDATION
428 West St. James Place
Second Floor
Chicago, Illinois 60614
USA
Tel: 1 800 843 2256

NATIONAL OSTEOPOROSIS
FOUNDATION
1150 17th Street
Suite 500
Washington, DC 20036
USA
Tel: 1 800 223 9994

NATIONAL PSORIASIS FOUNDATION
Suite 200
6415 South West Canyon Court
Portland, Oregon 97221
USA
Tel: 1 503 297 1545

HERBALISM

Australasia

NATIONAL HERBALISTS
ASSOCIATION OF AUSTRALIA
Suite 305, BST House
3 Smail Street
Broadway
New South Wales 2007
Australia
Tel: 61 2 211 6437
Fax: 61 2 211 6452

Europe

BRITISH HERBAL MEDICINE
ASSOCIATION
1 Wickham Road
Boscombe
Bournemouth
Dorset BH7 6JX
Great Britain
Tel: 44 1202 433691

THE HERB SOCIETY
Deddington Hill Farm
Warmington
Banbury
Oxon OX17 1XB
Great Britain
Tel: 44 1295 692900

NATIONAL INSTITUTE OF
MEDICAL HERBALISTS
56 Longbrook Street
Exeter
Devon EX4 6AH
Great Britain
Tel: 44 1392 426022

SCHOOL OF HERBAL
MEDICINE/PHYTOTHERAPY
Bucksteep Manor
Bodle Street Green
Near Hailsham
Sussex BN27 4RJ
Great Britain
Tel: 44 1323 834 800
Fax: 44 1323 834 801

North America

AMERICAN BOTANICAL COUNCIL
PO Box 201660
Austin
Texas 78720-1660
USA
Tel: 1 512 331 1924

AMERICAN HERBALISTS GUILD
PO Box 1683
Soquel
California 95073
USA

HOMEOPATHY

Australasia

AUSTRALIAN HOMEOPATHIC
ASSOCIATION
11 Landsborough Terrace
Toowong 4006
Australia
Tel/Fax: 61 7 3371 7245
e-mail: vikiwill@powerup.com.au

AUSTRALIAN INSTITUTE
OF HOMEOPATHY
21 Bulah Heights
Berdwra Heights
New South Wales 2082
Australia

NEW ZEALAND INSTITUTE OF
CLASSICAL HOMEOPATHY
PO Box 7232
Wellesley Street
Auckland
New Zealand
e-mail: jwinston@actrix.gen.nz

Europe

BRITISH HOMOEOPATHIC
ASSOCIATION
27A Devonshire Street
London W1N 1RJ
Great Britain
Tel: 44 207 935 2163

CENTRE D'ETUDES
Homéopathiques de France
228 Boulevard Raspail
75014 Paris
France
Tel: 33 143 207896

FACULTY OF HOMEOPATHY
Hahnemann House
2 Powis Place
London WC1N 3HT
Great Britain
Tel: 44 207 837 9469

SOCIÉTÉ MÉDICAL DE
BIOTHÉRAPIE
62 rue Beaubourg
75003 Paris
France
Tel: 33 143 346000

SOCIETY OF HOMOEOPATHS
2 Artisan Road
Northampton NN1 4HU
Great Britain
Tel: 44 1604 21400
Fax: 44 1604 22622

North America

HOMEOPATHIC ASSOCIATION
OF NATUROPATHIC
PHYSICIANS (HANP)
PO Box 69565
Portland
Oregon 97201
USA
Tel: 1 503 795 0579

NATIONAL CENTER FOR
HOMEOPATHY
801 North Fairfax Street
Suite 306
Alexandria
Virginia 22314
USA
Tel: 1 703 548 7790
Fax: 1 703 548 7792
e-mail: nch@igc.org

NORTH AMERICAN SOCIETY OF
HOMEOPATHS (NASH)
2024 S. Dearborn Street
Seattle
Washington 98144-2912
USA
Tel: 1 206 720 7000
Fax: 1 206 329 5684
e-mail: NashInfo@aol.com
Website: www.homeopathy.org

NUTRITION

Europe

THE BRITISH NATUROPATHIC
ASSOCIATION
Frazer House
6 Netherhall Gardens
London NW3 5RR
Great Britain
Tel: 44 207 435 7830

EATING DISORDERS ASSOCIATION
Sackville Place
44 Magdalen Street
Norwich NR3 1JU
Great Britain
Helpline: 44 1603 621414
Fax: 44 1603 664915
Website: www.gurney.org.uk/eda/

VEGETARIAN SOCIETY
Parkdale
Dunham Road
Altrincham
Cheshire WA14 4QG
Great Britain
Tel: 44 161 928 4QG
Fax: 44 161 926 9182

North America

AMERICAN ASSOCIATION OF
NUTRITION CONSULTANTS
1641 East Sunset Road,
Apt B-117
Las Vegas
Nevada 89119
USA
Tel: 1 709 361 1132

AMERICAN DIETETICS
ASSOCIATION
216 West Jackson Boulevard
Apt 800
Chicago
Illinois 60606-6995
USA
Tel: 1 800 877 1600

EATING DISORDERS AWARENESS
AND PREVENTION
603 Steward Street
Suite 8013
Seattle
Washington 98101
USA
Tel: 1 206 382 3587

NORTH AMERICAN VEGETARIAN
SOCIETY
PO Box 72
Dolgeville
New York NY 13329
USA
Tel: 1 518 568 7970

Index

Contributors

NAOMI CRAFT, Bsc., MBBS, MRCGP, qualified in 1988 and is now a general practitioner in London. A regular contributor to self-help books, she has also written for magazines and newspapers and has appeared on television and radio. In 1996 she received an award for excellence from the Medical Journalists' Association.

JOSIE DRAKE, ITEC, Phys.ETh., AIPTI, LTPhys., is a highly qualified therapist who specializes in teaching massage, aromatherapy, diet nutrition, and stress management. She has also worked at Stoke Mandeville Hospital and was acclaimed the 1997 National Health and Beauty's Community Therapist of the Year.

DR. FIONA DRY, MBBS, MRCGP, DSMSA, MFHom. is a general practitioner and homeopath who is based in Leighton Buzzard, Bedfordshire, England. She also works as a sports physician for the Badminton Association of England, treating its elite athletes.

PENELOPE ODY is a member of the National Institute of Medical Herbalists and a Fellow of the Herb Society, and ran her own herbal practice in Buckinghamshire for 12 years. She has written books on herbal medicine and home remedies, and lectures widely on these themes.

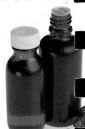

C. NORMAN SHEALY, M.D., Ph.D., is founding President of the American Holistic Medical Association and of the Shealy Center, America's foremost alternative-medicine clinic.

MICHAEL VAN STRATEN is a registered naturopath, osteopath, and acupuncturist and a former governor of the British College of Naturopathy and Osteopathy. The author of many books on the subject of nutrition and natural health, he is also a health journalist writing for newspapers and magazines, and a prolific radio and TV broadcaster. He also runs his own naturopathy practices in London and Buckinghamshire.